Sex Steroid Hormones - Impact on Reproductive Physiology

Edited by Courtney Marsh

Published in London, United Kingdom

Sex Steroid Hormones - Impact on Reproductive Physiology
http://dx.doi.org/10.5772/intechopen.1004954
Edited by Courtney Marsh

Contributors
Angel Benny Wisan, Ei Terasawa, Frederick Yeboah Obese, Godspower Onyeso, I Gusti Agung Ngurah Agung Sentosa, Japheth David, Joshua Salifu Wuntimah Mogre, Juliana Bicca, Kenneth P. Roberts, Kyle C. Schuppe, Menizibeya Welcome, Michael Egwu, Ryan J. Adam, Sadat Salifu, Stephen A. Osei

First published in London, United Kingdom, 2025 by IntechOpen
IntechOpen is the global imprint of INTECHOPEN LIMITED, registered in England and Wales, registration number: 11086078, 167-169 Great Portland Street, London, W1W 5PF, United Kingdom

For EU product safety concerns: IN TECH d.o.o., Prolaz Marije Krucifikse Kozulić 3, 51000 Rijeka, Croatia, info@intechopen.com or visit our website at intechopen.com.

British Library Cataloguing-in-Publication Data
A catalogue record for this book is available from the British Library

Sex Steroid Hormones - Impact on Reproductive Physiology
Edited by Courtney Marsh
p. cm.
Print ISBN 978-1-83634-023-2
Online ISBN 978-1-83634-022-5
eBook (PDF) ISBN 978-1-83634-024-9

Meet the editor

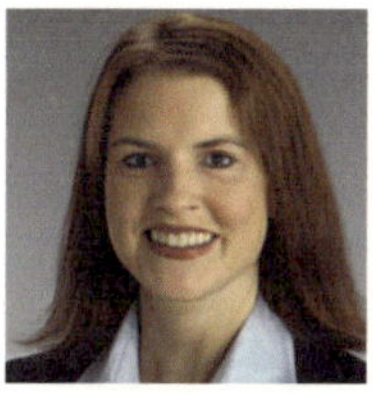

Dr. Courtney Marsh is certified by the American Board of Obstetrics and Gynecology with a subcertification in reproductive endocrinology. She completed a fellowship at the University of Michigan. She earned her medical degree from the University of Kansas School of Medicine and completed her residency at Emory University. Dr. Marsh is passionate about helping couples get pregnant. She has published over fifty peer-reviewed journal articles and has authored multiple book chapters on reproductive physiology and infertility. Dr. Marsh has a busy clinical practice at the University of Kansas Health System, helping patients build families and manage complex reproductive hormonal issues.

Contents

Preface

Sex Steroid Hormones – Impact on Reproductive Physiology covers progestins, androgens and estrogens and their regulation.

Our first section, "Sex Steroid Hormone Regulation," looks at the production and activity of sex steroid hormones and how they are regulated. Chapter 1, "Regulation of GnRH Release by Neuroestrogens in Non-human Primates", delves into the hypothalamic control of sex steroid activity. Focusing on non-human primates, the hypothalamic-pituitary-gonadal axis is explained in detail. In chapter 2, "Sex Hormone Binding Globulin: Multiple Modes of Action in Sex Steroid Hormone Signaling", the authors focus on how the glycoprotein primarily produced by the liver binds to sex steroid hormones and regulates bioavailability and activity. In chapter 3, "Sex Steroid Hormone Dynamics in Reproduction in Sheep", the author uses an animal model to explore negative and positive feedback and regulation of the hypothalamic-pituitary-gonadal axis.

Section 2 focuses on progestins with the chapter "Role of Progestins in Reproduction". Progestins are crucial in maintaining pregnancy and supporting the luteal phase after ovulation. The authors also explore the broader role of progestins, as they are central to the regulation of reproduction and contraception.

Section 3 focuses on androgens with the chapter "Disorder-Related Sex Steroid Hormonal Production: Polycystic Ovarian Syndrome". Polycystic ovarian syndrome is characterized by hyperandrogenism, and this chapter explores the role of sex steroid hormone production in the dysregulation. The pathophysiology for polycystic ovarian syndrome is complex, involving increased androgens, progesterone deficiency and imbalance of luteinizing and follicle-stimulating hormones.

Section 4 focuses on estrogens, and the chapter "Reproductive Landmarks and Lipedema: Lessons to be Learned about Women Hormones throughout Life" examines the complex interplay between lipedema and estrogen. Lipedema is a chronic condition characterized by abnormal accumulations of adipose tissue, particularly in the extremities. As the condition is predominantly in women and worsens with hormonal changes, the role of estrogen and its possible impact on the severity and progression of lipedema is explored.

Overall, the book looks at all sex steroid hormones, their regulation and their impact on reproductive physiology. We hope you enjoy the book and have a better understanding of the complex role sex steroid hormones have on reproduction and overall health after reading.

Courtney Marsh
University of Kansas Medical Center,
Kansas City, United States of America

Section 1

Sex Steroid Hormone Regulation

Chapter 1

Regulation of GnRH Release by Neuroestrogens in Non-human Primates

Ryan J. Adam and Ei Terasawa

Abstract

This chapter summarizes recent progress in reproductive neuroendocrinology in rhesus monkeys as a model for humans. First, to characterize properties of primate GnRH neurons, GnRH neurons are isolated from rhesus monkey embryos and cultured, and human GnRH neurons are generated from induced pluripotent human stem cells. Results from cultured GnRH neurons indicate that exposure to estradiol rapidly stimulates firing activity, increases Ca^{2+} oscillations, synchronization of Ca^{2+} oscillations among GnRH neurons, and estrogen-induced GnRH release. Second, we describe a series of findings *in vivo*, showing that neuroestrogens, locally synthesized and released within the hypothalamus, play an important role in reproduction: Blocking neuroestrogens synthesis alters the pulsatility of gonadotropin releasing hormone (GnRH) release, and the estradiol-induced GnRH/LH-surge in ovariectomized females. Third, neuroestrogen recapitulates the rapid estrogen action in the brain. Collectively, these findings indicate importance of neuroestrogens in regulation of the HPG-axis.

Keywords: neuroestrogen, GnRH neuron, primates, hypothalamus, cell culture

1. Introduction

Ovarian derived estrogens play a central role in the hypothalamo-pituitary-gonadal (HPG) axis and female reproductive function. During early to mid-follicular phase of the ovulatory cycle, when circulating estrogen levels are low, estrogens inhibit gonadotropin releasing hormone (GnRH) release from the hypothalamus, and thereby luteinizing hormone (LH) and follicle stimulating hormone (FSH) from the anterior pituitary gland (negative feedback effects). During late-follicular phase, however, an increase in circulating estrogens from the matured follicle facilitates release of GnRH, LH and FSH (positive feedback effects), resulting in ovulation. While the importance of ovarian estrogens in regulation of reproductive cycles is well recognized, the role of estrogens synthesized in the brain is less appreciated. In 1971, Naftolin et al. reported aromatase enzyme activity in the human brain by observing conversion of radioactively tagged androstenedione to estrone (E_1) and 17β-estradiol (E_2) in tissue homogenates of the median eminence in the hypothalamus, [1] suggesting the *de novo* synthesis of estrogens in the brain. Since then, the role of neuroestrogens in brain fuction has been studied in a wide variety of animals [2, 3]. The presence of aromatase enzyme that converts

IntechOpen

androstendione and testosterone to estrone and estradiol, respectively, is identified in cell bodies, axons, and axo-terminals of neurons in a variety of species including humans and non-human primates [4–6]. Hence, the term *neuroestrogen* was established to represent estrogens produced by neurons, and the role of neuroestrogens in the brain function has been investigated for over 50 years. For example, Lu and Brann et al., reported significant memory deficits and diminished astrocyte mediated neuroprotection in forebrain aromatase knock-out mice [7, 8]. Zhou et al. described that treatment of mice with aromatase inhibitor resulted in impaired hippocampus synaptic plasticity and cognitive deficits [9]. In the hypothalamus, the presence of aromatase mRNA and protein, as well as aromatase activity are described, and the significance of neuroestrogens in the hypothalamo-pituitary-gonadal-axis has been reported [6, 10–14]. We have been studying whether and how neuroestrogens are involving in regulation of GnRH release for some time. In this chapter we summarize our recent findings.

2. E_2 rapidly and directly stimulates GnRH release from GnRH neurons *in vitro*

Until ~25 years ago, it was widely believed that the genomic action of estrogens on GnRH neurons was indirectly mediated through other neurons or glia. This concept was based on the observation that nuclear estrogen receptor expression was absent in GnRH neurons [15]. We have made a breakthrough. Toward investigating GnRH regulation at the molecular and cellular levels we developed a primary cell culture system of GnRH neurons. Knowing GnRH neurons originate from the embryonic olfactory placode and migrate into the pre-optic area and hypothalamus during the early embryonic stage [16], we dissected out olfactory placode and the migratory pathway of GnRH neurons from time-mated monkey fetuses and cultured them [17]. Under the microscope GnRH neurons were easily identifiable, as they exhibited fusiform shape and there were no other type of neurons originating from the olfactory placode at this developmental stage. Using these GnRH neurons, we characterized electrophysiological properties and factors influencing GnRH neuronal activity. As such, it was a huge surprise for us to observe that estradiol induced rapid excitatory action

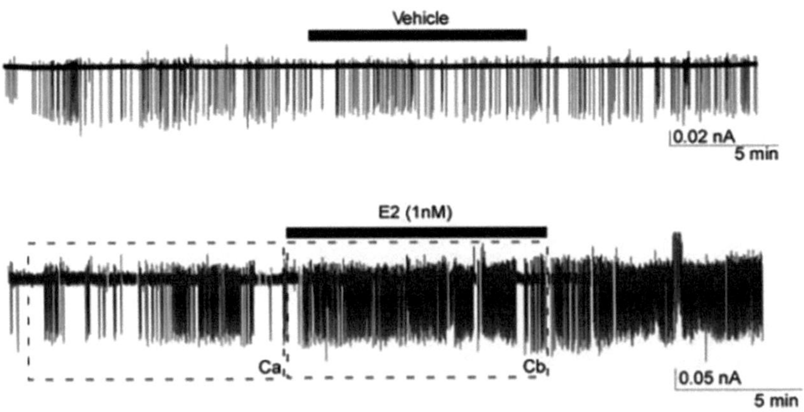

Figure 1.
Example showing the effects of vehicle (top) or estradiol (E_2, bottom) on single unit activity of GnRH neurons. Note that significant increases in firing activity are seen shortly after the start of exposure to 1 nM estradiol, but not vehicle. Figure adapted from Abe et al. [18].

when applied to cultured monkey GnRH neurons. In fact, when estradiol was directly applied to GnRH neurons, single unit firing activity with patch-clamp recording, and synchronization of intracellular calcium oscillations among GnRH neurons were dramatically increased [17, 18]. More specifically, exposure of GnRH neurons to estradiol (1 nM) for 10 minutes resulted in robust increases in firing frequency, as shown by **Figure 1** [18]. The latency of increased firing rate was 60 and 120 seconds after the estradiol application in the media, and the response lasted for as long as patch clamp seal integrity was maintained, up to 25 minutes, 15 minutes beyond removal of estradiol from the media [18]. Using Ca^{2+} imaging, we also found that application of 17β-estradiol (1 nM) to the culture media resulted in increased frequency of intracellular Ca^{2+} oscillations within minutes, and enhanced synchronization of Ca^{2+} pulses among GnRH neurons [19, 20], as illustrated by **Figure 2**. These observations clearly indicate estradiol induces a rapid, direct, excitatory action. Do these cells release the decapeptide GnRH in response to estradiol? To answer this question, we used a perifusion system in which media was continuously infused, while perifusates were collected at a 10-minute interval for several hours. As shown in **Figure 3**, we found that treatment with estradiol (1 nM) resulted in a significant increase in GnRH decapeptide release within 10 minutes and elevated GnRH release remained throughout the entire 20-minute estradiol treatment, and began returning to baseline levels approximately 30 minutes after estradiol removal. In contrast, vehicle treatment induced no effect [21]. These *in vitro* experiments demonstrate that estradiol rapidly stimulates

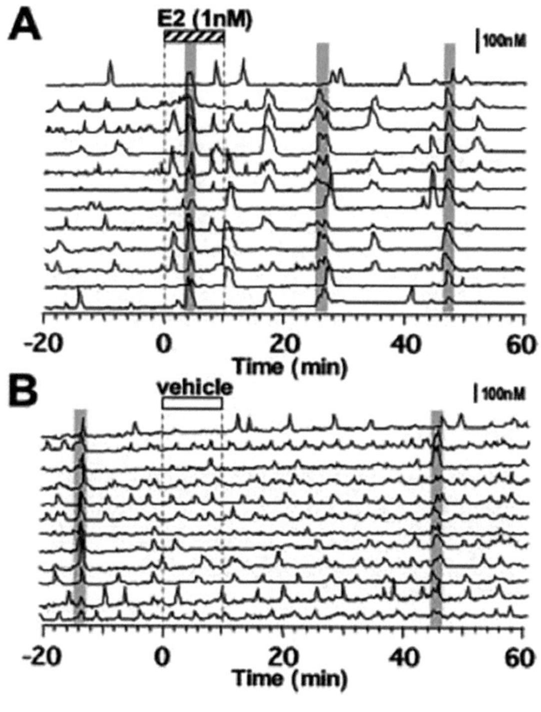

Figure 2.
Effects of estradiol (E_2, A) and vehicle (B) on Ca^{2+} oscillations and synchronization among cultured GnRH neurons. Each line represents the Ca^{2+} signal from a sigle GnRH neuron. Note that after the intial 20 min control recording, either E_2 or vehicle was infused for 10 min, and recording was continued an additional 60 min. Vertical gray bars indicate the synchronized Ca^{2+} increases among recorded GnRH neurons. Figure adapted from Abe et al. [19].

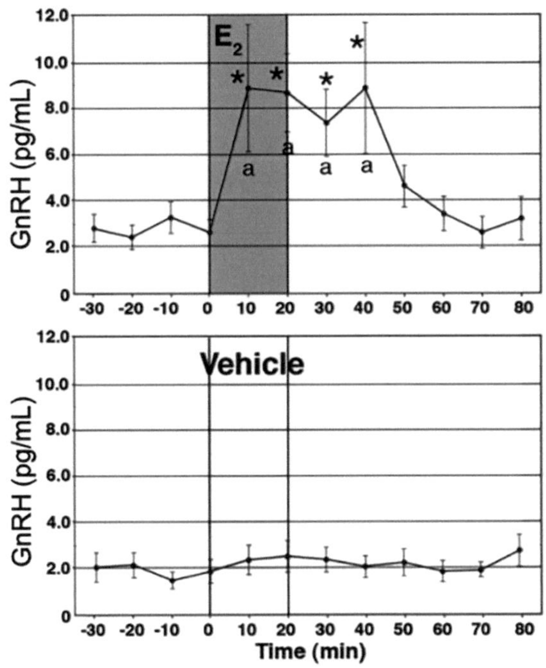

Figure 3.
In vitro *treatment of GnRH neurons with estradiol (E_2) for 20 min (top), but not vehicle (bottom), resulted in significant increases in GnRH release. The gray bar indicates E_2 treatment.* *$P < 0.05$ *versus before* E_2. *a,* $P < 0.05$ *versus vehicle at the corresponding time. Figure adapted from Noel et al. [21].*

firing activity, frequency of the intra-cellar Ca^{2+} oscillations, synchronization of Ca^{2+} oscillations among GnRH neurons, and decapeptide GnRH release.

3. Mechanisms of estrogen action in GnRH neurons *in vitro*

What is the mechanism initiating the rapid and direct estrogen action on GnRH neurons? We began to examine this question by treating cells with ICI182,780 (ICI), an ERα and ERβ receptor antagonist. Using patch clamp recording, we found that administration of ICI completely blocked estradiol-induced increases in firing activity [18], while failed to block estradiol-induced increases in intracellular Ca^{2+} oscillations and synchronization of Ca^{2+} oscillation among GnRH neurons [19]. Importantly, ICI failed to significantly attenuate estradiol-induced increases in GnRH release [21]. We next investigated possible estrogen action through ERα and ERβ by treating these cells with ERα and ERβ siRNA prior to E_2 treatment [20]. The results with qPCR indicated knockdown of respective receptor mRNA by >90% confirming the effectiveness of the treatment [20]. Results of intracellular Ca^{2+}imaging, however, indicate that, similar to ICI, siRNA knockdown failed to alter E_2-induced changes in intracellular Ca^{2+} activity [20]. Taken together, these findings indicate that rapid estrogen action resulting in alteration of intracellular Ca^{2+} oscillations and peptide release in GnRH neurons are independent of the mechanism mediated through ERα and ERβ. Interestingly, changes in cellular firing pattern, assessed by patch clamp recording, were sensitive to ICI, suggesting the presence of a mechanism for rapid excitatory estrogen action mediated through ERα and/or ERβ, which does not lead to rapid release of GnRH peptide.

DOI: http://dx.doi.org/10.5772/intechopen.1008513

Since rapid excitatory estrogen action resulting in GnRH release is not mediated through ERα or ERβ, how did estradiol induce its action on GnRH neurons? Toward approaching this question, we next investigated whether E_2 initiates its actions at the cell membrane, cytoplasm, and/or nucleus. We treated cells with estrogen dendrimer conjugate (EDC), which is unable to pass through the nuclear membrane. Administration of EDC, but not dendrimer conjugate itself as a control, induced similar effects as estradiol on Ca^{2+} imaging including significant increases in Ca^{2+} oscillations, and increased synchronous oscillations among cells [19]. Treatment of GnRH neurons with EDC also resulted in significant elevations in GnRH release [21]. The similar effects of EDC with those of E_2 suggest that the mechanism initiating E_2 action lies within the cytoplasm and/or cell membrane. We next applied estradiol-17 hemisuccinate BSA (E_2-BSA), which cannot cross the cell membrane. Upon treatment, we found that E_2-BSA induced significant elevations in GnRH release, although the increase in response to E_2-BSA was not as large, nor as long lasting as E_2 alone [21]. Collectively, the results from this series of experiments are interpreted to mean that (1) a significant portion of estrogen initiating its action, similar to the recent work of Faure et al. [22] occurs at the cell membrane levels of GnRH neurons, but a minor estrogen action may occur at cytoplasm, and (2) estradiol action at the cell membrane is responsible for stimulation of GnRH peptide release, because cell membrane impermeable estradiol resulted in stimulation of GnRH release.

Accordingly, we have hypothesized that the G protein-coupled receptor 30 (GPR30), a seven transmembrane G-protein receptor, mediates rapid E_2 action in GnRH neurons, as it has been reported that GPR30 mediates membrane action of estrogens in cancer cells [23]. Using RT-PCR we found that GPR30 mRNA is expressed in GnRH neurons in culture as well as in the hypothalamus of rhesus monkeys [21]. In addition, with immunostaining, we observed GPR30 positive expression in a subset of GnRH neurons in the rhesus monkey hypothalamus [21]. To investigate whether GPR30 is involved in rapid estrogen actions, we employed an siRNA knockdown approach similar to that we previously describe for ERα and ERβ. We found that while estradiol stimulated Ca^{2+}oscillations and synchronization among GnRH neurons in cells transfected with control siRNA, siRNA knockdown of GPR30 significantly attenuated, but did not eliminate, these changes [21]. We further examined whether GPR30 mediates rapid estrogen action by applying G1, a specific GPR30 agonist [24]. The results show that treatment of GnRH neurons with G1, but not vehicle, resulted in a significant increase in frequency of Ca^{2+} oscillations, similar to those seen with estradiol treatment [21], although G1 did not significantly affect synchronization of Ca^{2+} oscillations among GnRH neurons [21]. Moreover, G1 treatment facilitated GnRH release (unpublished observation). Taken together, these data are consistent with the hypothesis that E_2, through GPR30, imparts rapid stimulatory action on GnRH neurons.

siRNA knockdown of GPR30 partially, not completely, blocked effects of estradiol, suggesting the possible involvement of additional receptors in rapid estrogen action. We have examined the possible involvement of the receptor encoding diphenylacrylamide (STX). STX is an estrogenic compound and it has been shown to elicit effects similar to those with estrogens on energy metabolism, body temperature regulation, and reproduction, among others [25–27]. Moreover, the receptor for STX (STX-R) is located on the cell membrane, and differs from GPR30, ERα, and ERβ [25–28]. Importantly, STX dependent signaling, including response to the GABA agonist, baclofen, on patch clamp, is not affected by respective mouse knockouts of ERα, ERβ, and GPR30 receptors in POMC neurons in the arcuate nucleus of the hypothalamus [25–28]. Additionally, it has been demonstrated that STX-R is sensitive to

ICI [26]. Accordingly, we hypothesized that a portion of the E_2 effects we observed in cultured GnRH neurons are mediated through STX-R. We tested this possibility with a series of *in vitro* experiments. We found that STX treatment of GnRH neurons *in vitro* at 10 nM and 100 nM resulted in dose dependent GnRH release (**Figure 4**), and increased frequency and synchronizations of Ca^{2+} oscillations among GnRH neurons [29]. These effects were unaffected by siRNA knockdown of GPR30 but were blocked by treatment with ICI, consistent with other studies in which ICI blocked the effects of STX [25–28]. As a known downstream pathway of STX action is phospholipase

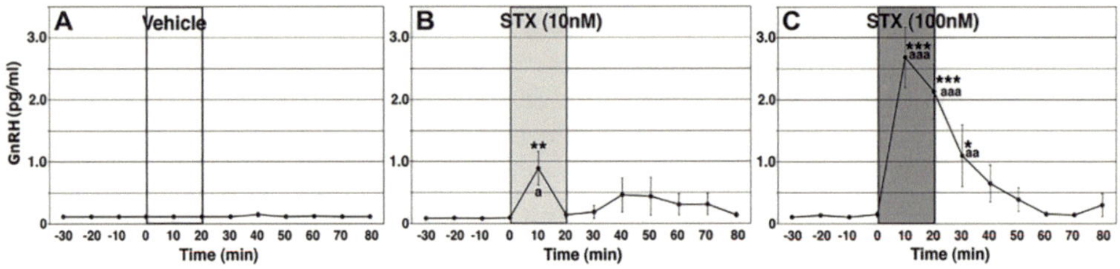

Figure 4.
Exposure of GnRH neurons to STX stimulated GnRH peptide release in vitro *in a dose dependent manner. After a 30-min control period, cells were exposed to vehicle (A), 10 nM STX (B), or 100 nM STX (C) and samples were collected for an additional 80 min.* *P < 0.05 *vs. before STX.* **P < 0.01 *vs. before STX.* ***P < 0.001 *vs. before STX.* ^{a}P < 0.05 *vs. vehicle.* ^{aa}P < 0.01 *vs. vehicle.* ^{aaa}P < 0.0001 *vs. vehicle. Figure adapted from Kenealy et al. [29].*

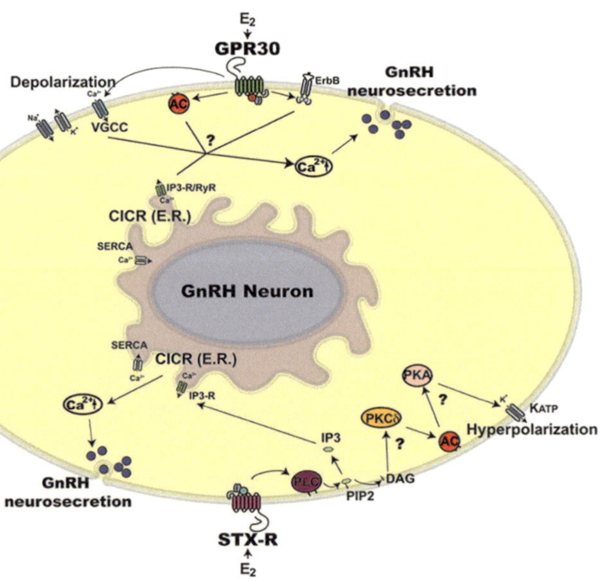

Figure 5.
This schematic illustration summarizes the mechanism of direct estradiol (E_2) action on the GnRH neuron. Estradiol (E_2) interacts with the membrane receptors GPR30 and STX-R, which ultimately lead to changes in intracellular Ca^{2+}oscillations. Question marks in the schema represent speculative mechanisms that require experimental validation. Abbreviations: GPR30, G protein coupled receptor 30; AC, adenylyl cyclase; CICR, calcium induced calcium release; DAG, diacylglycerol; ER, endoplasmic reticulum, ErbB, epidermal growth factor receptor; IP3, inositol triphosphate; IP3-R, inositol triphosphate receptor; KATP, ATP sensitive potassium channel; PIP2, phosphatidylinositol biphosphate; PKA, protein kinase A; PKCδ, Protein kinase C delta; PLC, phospholipase C; RyR, ryanodine receptor; SERCA, sarco/endoplasmic reticulum Ca^{2+} ATPase; STX-R, membrane estrogen receptor sensitive to STX; VGCC, voltage gated calcium channel. GPR30, G protein coupled estrogen receptor. Adapted from Kenealy et al. [30].

C (PLC), we examined whether PLC is involved in rapid estrogen action in GnRH neurons. We found that inhibition PLC with U73122 blocked STX effects. Because STX and GPR30 are both G protein-coupled receptors, we reasoned that application of the G protein coupled receptor blocker, pertussis toxin (PTX), would attenuate E_2 effects. Indeed, treatment with PTX blocked E_2 induced increases in Ca^{2+} oscillation frequency and percent of stimulated cells [21].

Collectively, this series of *in vitro* experiments established that E_2 rapidly stimulates intracellular Ca^{2+} activity, and GnRH peptide release in primate GnRH neurons, and these effects are mediated, in part, by membrane G-coupled receptors GPR30 and STX-R, [30] as summarized schematically in **Figure 5**. The results from *in vitro* experiments have a number of implications. First, rapid effects, occurring within minutes, after E_2 treatment indicate a non-genomic mechanism, as they do not require transcription and translation. Second, enhanced synchronization of Ca^{2+} pulses among GnRH neurons following E_2 treatments appears to be an underlying mechanism responsible for synchronization among GnRH neurons *in vivo*. Hence, it is possible that estradiol may modulate coordination of pulsatile GnRH release *in vivo*. Third, and most importantly, the presence of multiple estrogen receptor mechanism on GnRH neurons, rather than a single receptor mechanism, would facilitate a complex regulation of estrogen action.

4. Estradiol infusion into the stalk-median eminence stimulates release of GnRH and LH *in vivo*

In order to examine whether direct stimulatory effects of estradiol on GnRH release occur *in vivo*, we used a microdialysis method. This approach requires initial surgical placement of a cranial pedestal on the monkey skull [31]. With aid of an x-ray ventriculogram obtained during the cranial pedestal implantation surgery, a microdialysis probe is inserted into the stalk-median eminence (S-ME) through the cranial pedestal. **Figure 6** summarizes the setup for microdialysis experiments. This approach has several advantages for cellular study in non-human primates. First, we are able to deliver experimental agents to, and collect samples from, the S-ME, a small specific area in the bottom of the hypothalamus. This approach greatly reduces off-target effects of systemically administered agents while enabling us to directly modify GnRH secretory activity at neuroterminals, and to measure release of GnRH, rather than measuring LH as a surrogate GnRH marker. Second, microdialysis experiments can be performed in unanesthetized conscious monkeys, as they are well-trained in all aspects of the experimental set up. Third, samples can be obtained from the S-ME continuously at a time interval, such as 10–20 minutes, depending on the sensitivity of measurements, for up to a 12-hour period under our animal protocol.

Using the microdialysis method in ovariectomized (OVX) adult rhesus monkeys, we observed that EB infusion (100 nM) directly to the S-ME for 20 minutes stimulated GnRH release within 20 minutes [32]. Moreover, continuous S-ME infusion of EB for 4 and 7 hours, respectively, results in sustained increases in GnRH release and circulating LH concentration for several hours (**Figure 7A**) [33]. S-ME infusion of vehicle resulted in no changes (**Figure 7B**) [33]. In a separate experiment, subcutaneous injection of EB (50 μg/kg) lowered circulating LH for several hours (**Figure 7C**), [33] consistent with previous work from this lab [34], and the widely known negative feedback action of E_2 on GnRH and LH release. The results showing that infusion of EB directly to the S-ME, where GnRH neuroprocesses are

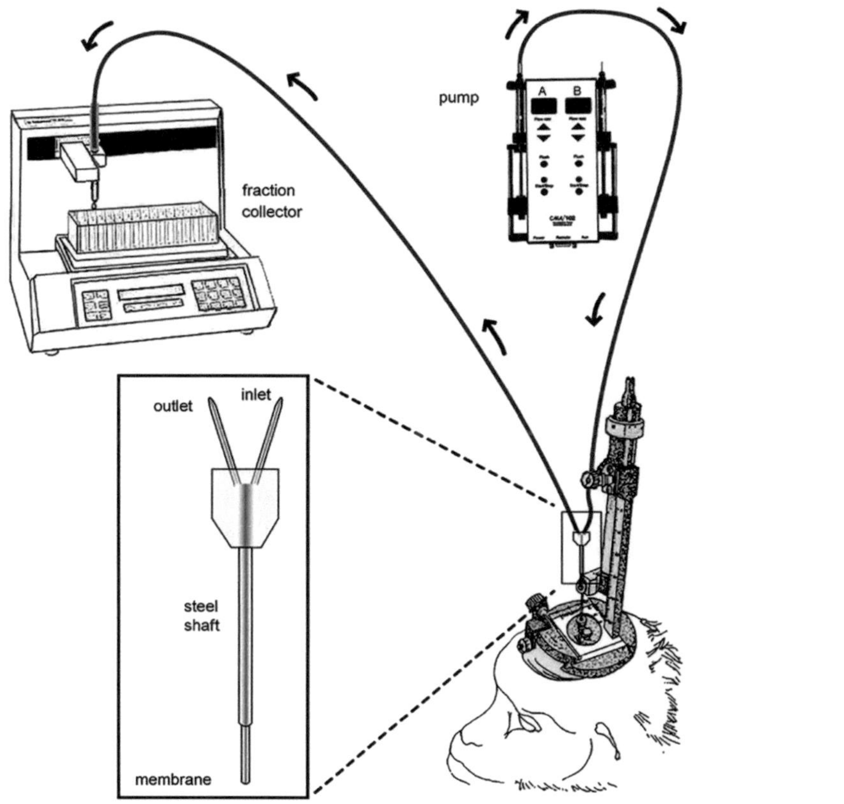

Figure 6.
Schematic illustration of the microdialysis method in the rhesus monkey. A custom-made microdialysis probe (insert) for the rhesus monkey was inserted into the stalk-median eminence of the hypothalamus through a permanently implanted cranial pedestal. The inlet of the probe is attached by tubing to a syringe pump that continuously infuses perfusion fluid, with or without experimental challenges. A probe outlet directs perfusate to a fraction collector for serial sampling and subsequent analysis. Arrows indicate the direction of fluid flow through the microdialysis probe and tubing. Figure adapted from Frost et al. [31].

concentrated, stimulates release of GnRH in adult, OVX, rhesus monkeys. These results are opposite from the effects of subcutaneously injected EB. Nevertheless, as local infusion of a small dose of estradiol mimics the role of neuroestradiol in the hypothalamus, we can speculate that neuroestradiol in the S-ME plays a role in regulation of GnRH release *in vivo*.

The rapid actions of estradiol on GnRH neurons *in vitro* lend support to the role of neuroestrogens as neurotransmitters [5]. The rapid stimulatory effects of estradiol on GnRH neurons observed *in vitro* experiments differs from canonical negative and positive feedback action of estradiol on GnRH release *in vivo*. Hence, similar rapid excitatory effects on GnRH release can be induced by electrical stimulation of the basal hypothalamus, we hypothesized that electrical stimulation also release estradiol. Indeed, application of electrical stimulation of the medial basal hypothalamus led to release of GnRH and estradiol in the S-ME *in vivo* (**Figure 8**), [32] while sham stimulation failed to induce any discernable increases in release of GnRH or estradiol [32].

Based on these results we reasoned that infusion of estradiol into the S-ME would elicit neuroestradiol release *in vivo*. In the experiment, we infused estradiol benzoate

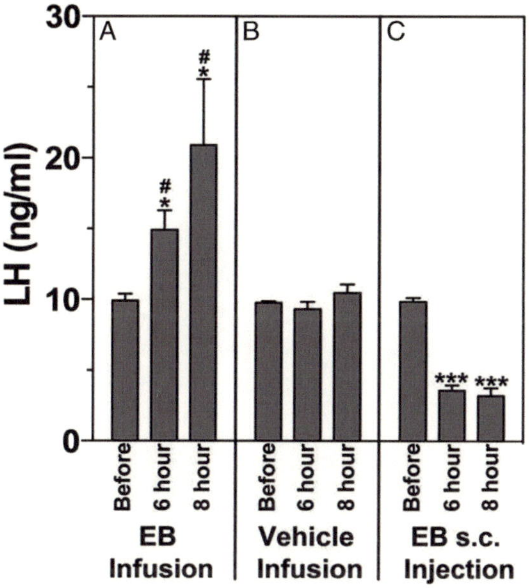

Figure 7.
*(A) Continuous EB infusion into the stalk-median eminence (S-ME) for 7-hour period stimulated prolonged release of circulating LH. (A) Serum samples were obtained before, 6, or 8 hours after the initiation of the 7-hour EB infusion. (B) Vehicle infusion into the S-ME did not change LH levels at the correspondent time. (C) For comparison, the effects of subcutaneous (s.c.) EB injection on LH release is shown. *P < 0.05 compared to before infusion. # P < 0.05 compared to corresponding time with vehicle treatment. ***P < 0.001 compared to before s.c. EB injection. Figure reproduced from Kenealy et al. [33].*

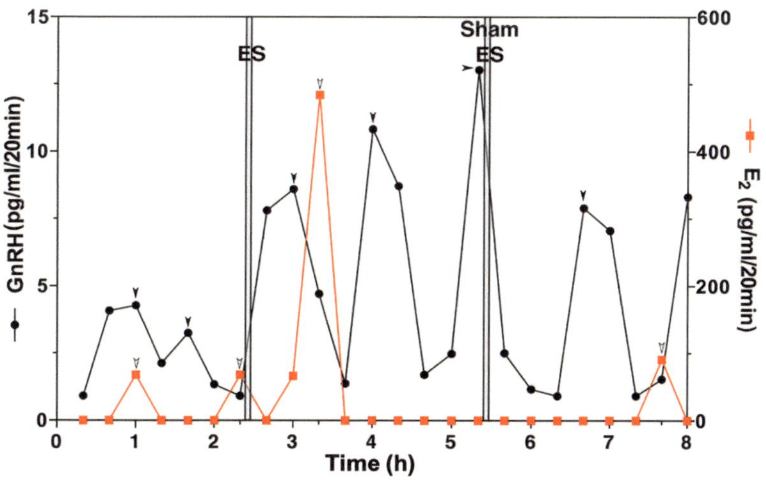

Figure 8.
Electrical stimulation (ES) of the basal hypothalamus, but not sham ES, elicits release of estradiol (E_2) into the stalk median eminence in conscious, adult, ovariectomized rhesus monkeys using microdialysis. Vertical bars indicate time period of ES or sham ES stimulation. Arrows mark peaks of estradiol and GnRH. Figure adapted from Kenealy et al. [32].

(EB) into the S-ME using microdialysis, and assessed changes in estradiol concentrations in dialysates. For measurements of estradiol concentrations, we employed liquid chromatography followed by mass spectrometry (LC/MS), instead of conventional immunologically based methods (i.e., EIA or RIA), because LC/MS differentiates

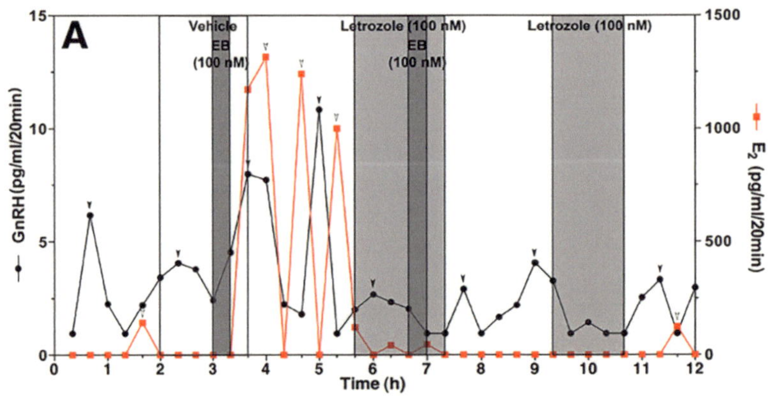

Figure 9.
Administration of estrogen benzoate (EB) by microdialysis to the S-ME of conscious, adult, OVX, rhesus macaques resulted in increases in GnRH release and E_2 release into the S-ME. Co-administration of the aromatase inhibitor letrozole with EB blocked these effects. Administration of letrozole alone had little effect. Dark gray bars represent times of EB infusion. Lighter gray bars represent times of letrozole infusion. White (unshaded) represent times of letrozole vehicle infusion. Figure adapted from Kenealy et al. [32].

between E_2 and EB molecules. The results indicate that EB infusion to the S-ME stimulated rapid release of estradiol as well as GnRH. Interestingly, the release of estradiol was pulsatile with peaks reaching over 1000 pg./mL. Moreover, infusion of EB in the S-ME in the presence of the aromatase inhibitor letrozole failed to increase in release of estradiol and GnRH (**Figure 9**). Collectively, these findings indicate importance of neuroestrogens locally synthesized in the basal hypothalamus in regulation of GnRH release.

5. Involvement of neuroestrogens in regulation of the LH surge

Based on the finding of neuroestrogens' role in GnRH pulsatility, we next investigated whether neuroestrogens play any role in the preovulatory GnRH/LH surge. As the GnRH/LH surge, similar to that seen during the late preovulatory phase, can be induced by a high dose of EB injection in ovariectomized females [32, 33], a group of ovariectomized females were implanted with capsules containing estradiol s.c., and two weeks later, a high dose of EB was injected in the presence or absence of the aromatase inhibitor letrozole. Results indicated that while in the absence of letrozole EB induced LH surges, in the presence of letrozole the EB induced-LH surge was significantly attenuated (**Figure 10**) [35]. Nevertheless, we needed to conduct another experiment, in which the role of hypothalamic neuroestrogens is directly examined, as aromatase enzyme is distributed widely throughout the body and letrozole was administered systemically. Accordingly, we applied letrozole to the S-ME directly and continuously for 6 hours, corresponding to hours 42–48 post-EB injection, the time when the expected EB-induced LH surge occurs. The results indicated that letrozole infusion in the S-ME greatly attenuated the LH surge (**Figure 11**) [35]. Together, these findings clearly indicate the significant role of neuroestrogen during the LH/GnRH surge. Collectively, we propose a modified concept on the positive feedback action of estradiol on GnRH/LH surge generation. In **Figure 12** we have included the role of hypothalamic kisspeptin/neurokinin B/dynorphin neurons, known as *KNDy neurons*, as they are the

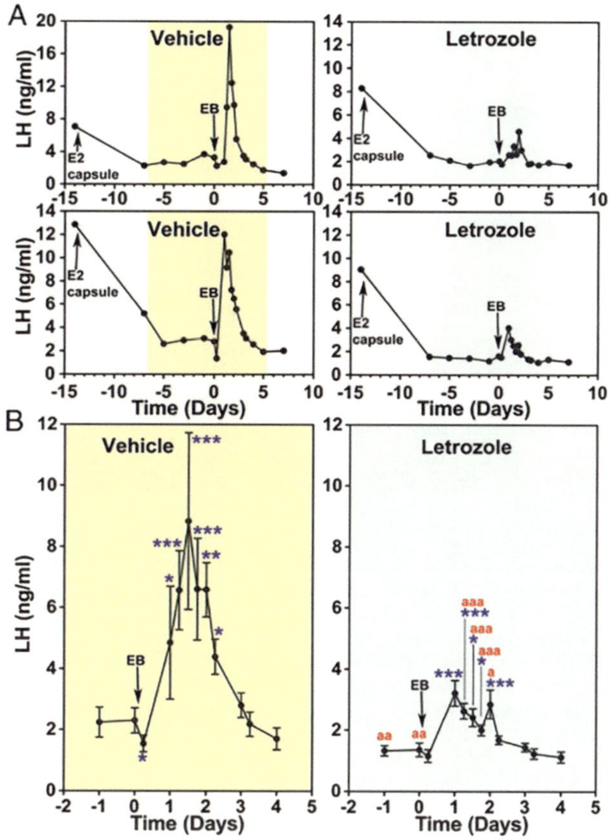

Figure 10.
Part A shows examples of circulating LH concentration from individual adult, OVX, rhesus macaques in which they received an s.c. E_2 secreting capsule two weeks prior to a single s.c. injection of EB (30 µg) to induce an LH surge. Daily vehicle or letrozole s.c. injections began 7 days prior to, and continued 5 days following the EB injection. Part B shows average LH surge curves averaged across treated animals. Observe the markedly attenuated curves in the letrozole treated animals. *P < 0.05 *vs. before EB treatment.* **P < 0.01 *vs. before EB treatment.* ***P < 0.001 *vs. before EB treatment.* [a]P < 0.05 *vs. corresponding time in vehicle treated group.* [aa]P < 0.01 *vs. corresponding time in vehicle treated group.* [aaa]P < 0.001 *vs. corresponding time in vehicle treated group. Figure adapted from Kenealy et al. [35].*

major target of circulating estradiol [36–38]. In sheep, rats, and mice, kisspeptin (K), neurokinin B (N), and dynorphin (Dy) colocalize in the same neurons and they are the direct upstream regulator of GnRH neurons. While kisspeptin and neurokinin B initiate a GnRH pulse, dynorphin terminates the pulse. Although the colocalization rate of kisspeptin, neurokinin B, and dynorphin in a single neuron is rare in primates, including humans, [39] the role of KNDy neurons in primates are very similar to those reported in sheep and rodents. For instance, our lab has demonstrated that administration of kisspeptin and senktide (a neurokinin B receptor agonist) to the S-ME via microdialysis, respectively induce rapid and pronounced release of GnRH in rhesus monkeys [40, 41]. KNDy neurons play important roles in sex steroid hormone feedback control. For example, ovariectomy has been shown to increase expression of kisspeptin and neurokinin B, and reintroduction of female gonadal steroid hormones a reduction, consistent with a negative feedback mechanism [42–45]. KNDy neurons also express female sex steroid hormone receptors including ERα. As we have detailed throughout this

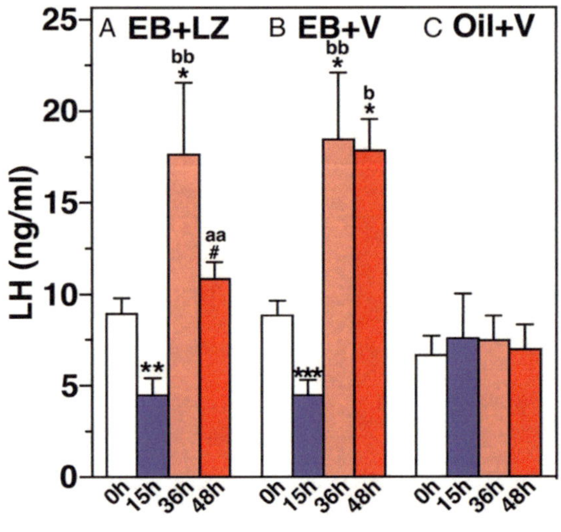

Figure 11.
We tested the effects of letrozole (LZ) administration via microdialysis to the hypothalamic S-ME on hours 42-48 h post administration of an s.c. EB injection, a time of anticipated LH surge. LH was measured from blood samples collected at the time of EB injection, 15 h, 36 h, and 48 h post EB injection. Shown are results for animals that received an (A) EB injection and letrozole infusion, (B) an EB injection with letrozole vehicle infusion, and (C) an EB vehicle (oil) injection with infusion of letrozole vehicle. **P < 0.01 vs. 0 h.* ***P < 0.01 vs. 0 h.* ****P < 0.001 vs. 0 h.* ^{b}*P < 0.05 vs. corresponding time in Oil+V group.* ^{bb}*P < 0.01 vs. corresponding time in Oil+V group.* ^{aa}*P < 0.01 vs. corresponding time in EB + V group.* $^{\#}$*P < 0.05 vs. 36 h time in EB + LZ group. Figure adapted from Kenealy et al. [35].*

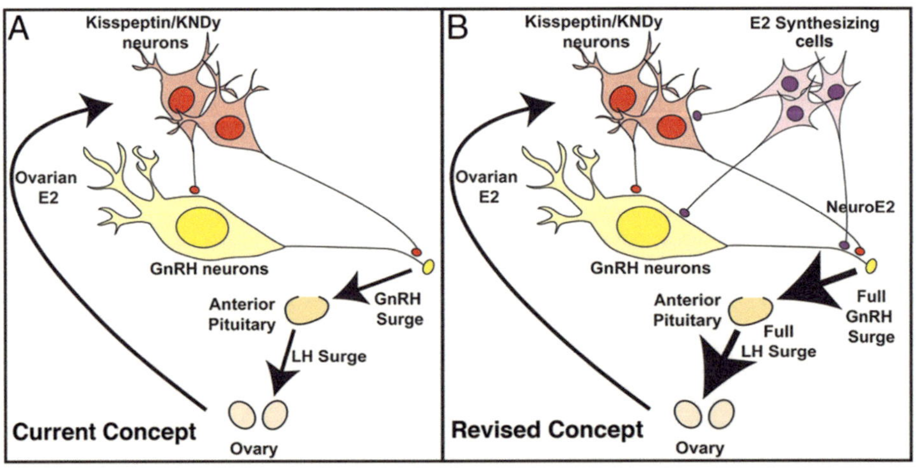

Figure 12.
(A) A schematic illustrating the historically traditional view of E_2 positive feedback in LH surge generation. In this view, ovarian E_2 reaches kisspeptin/KNDy neurons, that express ERα, are stimulated by E_2 and in turn, stimulate GnRH a surge leading to gonadotropin generation of an LH surge. Data from our laboratory suggests a revised concept (B). Ovarian E_2 stimulates kisspeptin/KNDy neurons and E_2 synthesis in the hypothalamus, which together stimulate release of a GnRH surge. It appears that stimulation of GnRH neurons by newly synthesized neuroestrogen is required to generate a full GnRH surge, and consequently, a full LH surge. Figure adapted from Kenealy et al. [35].

text, an underappreciated HPG axis regulatory mechanism is that circulating ovarian estradiol stimulates synthesis of hypothalamic neuroestrogens, which in turn, contributes to feedback loop regulation of the HPG axis.

6. Conclusion

We found, in adult, OVX, rhesus monkeys, that neuroestrogen, synthesized in the hypothalamus in an aromatase-dependent manner stimulates GnRH release when continuously administered for 20 minutes, 4 hours, and 7 hours, and appears required for generation of a full LH surge in our model of pre-ovulatory LH surge. We found that administration of EB to the hypothalamic S-ME induces synthesis of neuroestrogen locally. *In vitro*, we found treatment of GnRH neurons with E_2 to rapidly stimulate Ca^{2+} oscillations and intercellular synchronization and GnRH release. These effects are mediated, at least in part, through membrane G-couple protein receptors STX-R and GPR30. Collectively, these experiments, performed in non-human primates, and many virtually impossible to replicate in humans, position hypothalamic synthesis of neuroestrogen as a key regulator of GnRH release, and hence, the ovulatory cycle.

Acknowlegements

The authors thank the members of this laboratory for many years of their contributions. This work was supported by NIH grants (R01HD089495, R01HD011355, R01HD015433, R37HD043341) and made possible to perform by NIH support (P51OD011106) to the Wisconsin National Primate Research Center.

Conflict of interest

The authors have no conflicts to disclose.

Author details

Ryan J. Adam[1] and Ei Terasawa[1,2]*

1 University of Wisconsin-Madison, Wisconsin National Primate Research Center, Madison, WI, USA

2 Department of Pediatrics, University of Wisconsin-Madison, Wisconsin National Primate Research Center, Madison, WI, USA

*Address all correspondence to: terasawa@primate.wisc.edu

References

[1] Naftolin F, Ryan KJ, Petro Z. Aromatization of androstenedione by the diencephalon. The Journal of Clinical Endocrinology and Metabolism. 1971;**33**:368-370

[2] Brann DW, Lu Y, Wang J, Sareddy GR, Pratap UP, Zhang Q, et al. Brain-derived estrogen and neurological disorders. Biology (Basel). 2022;**11**:1698

[3] Remage-Healey L, Maidment NT, Schlinger BA. Forebrain steroid levels fluctuate rapidly during social interactions. Nature Neuroscience. 2008;**11**:1327-1334

[4] Naftolin F, Horvath TL, Jakab RL, Leranth C, Harada N, Balthazart J. Aromatase immunoreactivity in axon terminals of the vertebrate brain. An immunocytochemical study on quail, rat, monkey and human tissues. Neuroendocrinology. 1996;**63**:149-155

[5] Saldanha CJ, Remage-Healey L, Schlinger BA. Synaptocrine signaling: Steroid synthesis and action at the synapse. Endocrine Reviews. 2011;**32**:532-549

[6] Balthazart J, Foidart A, Surlemont C, Harada N. Neuroanatomical specificity in the co-localization of aromatase and estrogen receptors. Journal of Neurobiology. 1991;**22**:143-157

[7] Lu Y, Sareddy GR, Wang J, Zhang Q, Tang FL, Pratap UP, et al. Neuron-derived estrogen is critical for astrocyte activation and neuroprotection of the ischemic brain. The Journal of Neuroscience. 2020;**40**:7355-7374

[8] Lu Y, Sareddy GR, Wang J, Wang R, Li Y, Dong Y, et al. Neuron-derived estrogen regulates synaptic plasticity and memory. The Journal of Neuroscience. 2019;**39**:2792-2809

[9] Zhou L, Fester L, von Blittersdorff B, Hassu B, Nogens H, Prange-Kiel J, et al. Aromatase inhibitors induce spine synapse loss in the hippocampus of ovariectomized mice. Endocrinology. 2010;**151**:1153-1160

[10] MacLusky NJ, Naftolin F, Goldman-Rakic PS. Estrogen formation and binding in the cerebral cortex of the developing rhesus monkey. Proceedings of the National Academy of Sciences of the United States of America. 1986;**83**:513-516

[11] Flores F, Naftolin F, Ryan KJ. Aromatization of androstenedione and testosterone by rhesus monkey hypothalamus and limbic system. Neuroendocrinology. 1973;**11**:177-182

[12] Beyer C, Tramonte R, Hutchison RE, Sharp PJ, Barker PJ, Huskisson NS, et al. Aromatase-immunoreactive neurons in the adult female chicken brain detected using a specific antibody. Brain Research Bulletin. 1994;**33**:583-588

[13] Sasano H, Takashashi K, Satoh F, Nagura H, Harada N. Aromatase in the human central nervous system. Clinical Endocrinology. 1998;**48**:325-329

[14] Shen P, Campagnoni CW, Kampf K, Schlinger BA, Arnold AP, Campagnoni AT. Isolation and characterization of a zebra finch aromatase cDNA: in situ hybridization reveals high aromatase expression in brain. Brain Research. Molecular Brain Research. 1994;**24**:227-237

[15] Shivers BD, Harlan RE, Morrell JI, Pfaff DW. Absence of oestradiol

concentration in cell nuclei of LHRH-immunoreactive neurones. Nature. 1983;**304**:345-347

[16] Schwanzel-Fukuda M, Pfaff DW. The migration of luteinizing hormone-releasing hormone (LHRH) neurons from the medial olfactory placode into the medial basal forebrain. Experientia. 1990;**46**:956-962

[17] Terasawa E, Schanhofer WK, Keen KL, Luchansky L. Intracellular Ca(2+) oscillations in luteinizing hormone-releasing hormone neurons derived from the embryonic olfactory placode of the rhesus monkey. The Journal of Neuroscience. 1999;**19**:5898-5909

[18] Abe H, Terasawa E. Firing pattern and rapid modulation of activity by estrogen in primate luteinizing hormone releasing hormone-1 neurons. Endocrinology. 2005;**146**:4312-4320

[19] Abe H, Keen KL, Terasawa E. Rapid action of estrogens on intracellular calcium oscillations in primate luteinizing hormone-releasing hormone-1 neurons. Endocrinology. 2008;**149**:1155-1162

[20] Kenealy BP, Keen KL, Terasawa E. Rapid action of estradiol in primate GnRH neurons: The role of estrogen receptor alpha and estrogen receptor beta. Steroids. 2011;**76**:861-866

[21] Noel SD, Keen KL, Baumann DI, Filardo EJ, Terasawa E. Involvement of G protein-coupled receptor 30 (GPR30) in rapid action of estrogen in primate LHRH neurons. Molecular Endocrinology. 2009;**23**:349-359

[22] Faure MC, Corona R, Roomans C, Lenfant F, Foidart JM, Cornil CA. Role of membrane estrogen receptor alpha on the positive feedback of estrogens on Kisspeptin and GnRH neurons. eNeuro. 2024;**11**:1-17

[23] Filardo EJ, Thomas P. GPR30: A seven-transmembrane-spanning estrogen receptor that triggers EGF release. Trends in Endocrinology and Metabolism. 2005;**16**:362-367

[24] Bologa CG, Revankar CM, Young SM, Edwards BS, Arterburn JB, Kiselyov AS, et al. Virtual and biomolecular screening converge on a selective agonist for GPR30. Nature Chemical Biology. 2006;**2**:207-212

[25] Qiu J, Bosch MA, Tobias SC, Krust A, Graham SM, Murphy SJ, et al. A G-protein-coupled estrogen receptor is involved in hypothalamic control of energy homeostasis. The Journal of Neuroscience. 2006;**26**:5649-5655

[26] Qiu J, Ronnekleiv OK, Kelly MJ. Modulation of hypothalamic neuronal activity through a novel G-protein-coupled estrogen membrane receptor. Steroids. 2008;**73**:985-991

[27] Roepke TA, Qiu J, Bosch MA, Ronnekleiv OK, Kelly MJ. Cross-talk between membrane-initiated and nuclear-initiated oestrogen signalling in the hypothalamus. Journal of Neuroendocrinology. 2009;**21**:263-270

[28] Roepke TA, Bosch MA, Rick EA, Lee B, Wagner EJ, Seidlova-Wuttke D, et al. Contribution of a membrane estrogen receptor to the estrogenic regulation of body temperature and energy homeostasis. Endocrinology. 2010;**151**:4926-4937

[29] Kenealy BP, Keen KL, Ronnekleiv OK, Terasawa E. STX, a novel nonsteroidal estrogenic compound, induces rapid action in primate GnRH neuronal calcium dynamics and peptide release. Endocrinology. 2011;**152**:3182-3191

[30] Kenealy BP, Terasawa E. Rapid direct action of estradiol in GnRH neurons:

Findings and implications. Frontiers in Endocrinology (Lausanne). 2011;**2**:106

[31] Frost SI, Keen KL, Levine JE, Terasawa E. Microdialysis methods for in vivo neuropeptide measurement in the stalk-median eminence in the rhesus monkey. Journal of Neuroscience Methods. 2008;**168**:26-34

[32] Kenealy BP, Kapoor A, Guerriero KA, Keen KL, Garcia JP, Kurian JR, et al. Neuroestradiol in the hypothalamus contributes to the regulation of gonadotropin releasing hormone release. The Journal of Neuroscience. 2013;**33**:19051-19059

[33] Kenealy BP, Keen KL, Garcia JP, Richter DJ, Terasawa E. Prolonged infusion of estradiol benzoate into the stalk median eminence stimulates release of GnRH and kisspeptin in ovariectomized female rhesus macaques. Endocrinology. 2015;**156**:1804-1814

[34] Mizuno M, Terasawa E. Search for neural substrates mediating inhibitory effects of oestrogen on pulsatile luteinising hormone-releasing hormone release in vivo in ovariectomized female rhesus monkeys (Macaca mulatta). Journal of Neuroendocrinology. 2005;**17**:238-245

[35] Kenealy BP, Keen KL, Garcia JP, Kohlenberg LK, Terasawa E. Obligatory role of hypothalamic neuroestradiol during the estrogen-induced LH surge in female ovariectomized rhesus monkeys. Proceedings of the National Academy of Sciences of the United States of America. 2017;**114**:13804-13809

[36] Goodman RL, Herbison AE, Lehman MN, Navarro VM. Neuroendocrine control of gonadotropin-releasing hormone: Pulsatile and surge modes of secretion. Journal of Neuroendocrinology. 2022;**34**:e13094

[37] Terasawa E, Kenealy BP. Neuroestrogen, rapid action of estradiol, and GnRH neurons. Frontiers in Neuroendocrinology. 2012;**33**:364-375

[38] Stevenson H, Bartram S, Charalambides MM, Murthy S, Petitt T, Pradeep A, et al. Kisspeptin-neuron control of LH pulsatility and ovulation. Frontiers in Endocrinology (Lausanne). 2022;**13**:951938

[39] Hrabovszky E, Sipos MT, Molnar CS, Ciofi P, Borsay BA, Gergely P, et al. Low degree of overlap between kisspeptin, neurokinin B, and dynorphin immunoreactivities in the infundibular nucleus of young male human subjects challenges the KNDy neuron concept. Endocrinology. 2012;**153**:4978-4989

[40] Garcia JP, Guerriero KA, Keen KL, Kenealy BP, Seminara SB, Terasawa E. Kisspeptin and neurokinin B signaling network underlies the pubertal increase in GnRH release in female rhesus monkeys. Endocrinology. 2017;**158**:3269-3280

[41] Garcia JP, Keen KL, Kenealy BP, Seminara SB, Terasawa E. Role of Kisspeptin and neurokinin B signaling in male rhesus monkey puberty. Endocrinology. 2018;**159**:3048-3060

[42] Rometo AM, Krajewski SJ, Voytko ML, Rance NE. Hypertrophy and increased kisspeptin gene expression in the hypothalamic infundibular nucleus of postmenopausal women and ovariectomized monkeys. The Journal of Clinical Endocrinology and Metabolism. 2007;**92**:2744-2750

[43] Smith JT, Cunningham MJ, Rissman EF, Clifton DK, Steiner RA. Regulation of Kiss1 gene expression

in the brain of the female mouse. Endocrinology. 2005;**146**:3686-3692

[44] Smith JT, Clay CM, Caraty A, Clarke IJ. KiSS-1 messenger ribonucleic acid expression in the hypothalamus of the ewe is regulated by sex steroids and season. Endocrinology. 2007;**148**:1150-1157

[45] Moore AM, Coolen LM, Porter DT, Goodman RL, Lehman MN. KNDy cells revisited. Endocrinology. 2018;**159**:3219-3234

Chapter 2

Sex Hormone Binding Globulin: Multiple Modes of Action in Sex Steroid Hormone Signaling

Kyle C. Schuppe and Kenneth P. Roberts

Abstract

Human Sex Hormone Binding Globulin (SHBG) is a homodimeric glycoprotein expressed primarily in the liver and secreted into the blood. An ortholog of SHBG, named Androgen Binding Protein (ABP), is expressed in Sertoli cells of murine species and secreted into the lumen of the seminiferous tubule and interstitial compartment of the testis. SHBG and ABP bind androgens and estradiol with highest affinity for androgens. In this review we examine the functions of SHBG/ABP, such as its role in steroid binding and transport, effect on the levels of free androgens in the blood, and its interaction with cell surface receptors for facilitated androgen uptake and receptor mediated signaling. The correlation between SHBG levels in blood and various disease states in humans, such as type-2 diabetes and metabolic syndrome, are also discussed. A germ cell-specific form raises questions about a role for SHBG in germ cell function and fertilization. The potential roles of SHBG/ABP in mammalian physiology are multiple and the differences between human and murine SHBG/ABP biology are striking and may lead to new areas of new investigation.

Keywords: sex hormone binding globulin, SHBG, androgen binding protein, ABP, testosterone, estrogen, testis

1. Introduction

Human Sex Hormone Binding Globulin (SHBG) is a homodimeric glycoprotein encoded by the SHBG gene on chromosome 17p13.1. The gene is predominantly expressed in the liver, and SHBG is secreted into the blood. In murine species, an ortholog of SHBG, named Androgen Binding Protein (ABP), is expressed primarily in Sertoli cells and secreted both into the lumen of the seminiferous tubule and the interstitium of the testis. SHBG and ABP bind androgens with high affinity. They also bind to estradiol and other steroid hormones. SHBG/ABP has been implicated in steroid binding and transport, and in affecting the levels of free androgens in the blood. SHBG has also been implicated in androgen uptake by cells and as a signaling molecule with cell surface receptors on target cells. SHBG levels in blood have been shown to correlate with various disease states such as type-2 diabetes and metabolic syndrome. A germ cell-specific form has been identified in the human testis, raising questions about a role for SHBG in germ cell function and fertilization. Clearly, the potential roles of SHBG and ABP are multiple. The objective of this review is to summarize the experimentally confirmed actions of SHBG/ABP, highlighting informative differences between human and murine SHBG biology, and to suggest areas of new inquiry. In this review, we will refer to ABP as murine SHBG, in accordance with the nomenclature used by the National Center for Biotechnology Information (NCBI).

2. Structure of SHBG

A cDNA encoding rat SHBG was published in 1985, followed in 1987 by the isolation of cDNAs encoding human SHBG in three independent laboratories [1–5]. The gene for human SHBG was subsequently cloned and found to contain 8 exons encoding a 402 amino acid precursor protein, which is cleaved to remove a 29 amino acid leader sequence (**Figure 1**) [8, 9]. The orthologous murine genes encoding SHBG have also been cloned and characterized and were shown to encode an 8 exon transcript that is expressed in the testis [10, 11]. These initial studies also revealed several potential splice variants of the SHBG mRNA involving an alternative first exon and exons 7 and 8. The domains responsible for steroid binding and dimerization are encoded within exons 3 and 4 [12, 13]. The region responsible for binding of SHBG to the putative SHBG receptor (R_{SHBG}) is mediated by a decapeptide sequence encoded within exon 3 (**Figure 1**) [14].

Crystal structure analysis and site-directed mutagenesis studies have revealed that human SHBG is a homodimer with each subunit containing a functional steroid-binding site [13, 15]. Each SHBG monomer comprises two laminin G-like (LG) domains, with the N-terminal LG domain containing both the steroid binding site and the regions that interact in dimerization [16]. LG domains have a spherical shape and consist of two regions, each containing 7 antiparallel β-sheets, packed on top of each other [13]. A subset of these strands, 4 in each set of antiparallel β-sheets, form a jellyroll motif [17]. A highly conserved disulfide bridge is formed between C164 and C188 at the C-terminus of the domain. The steroid ligand binds close to the center of the N-terminal LG domain, intercalating into the hydrophobic core between two β-sheets. The crystal structure suggests that dimerization occurs by interaction of β-strand 7 in one monomer with β-strand 10 in the other and this has been confirmed by mutation studies [13, 15]. SHBG contains an 0-linked glycan attached to Thr7 and two N-linked chains in the C-terminal LG-domain at Asn351 and Asn367 (**Figure 1**) [18]. N-glycosylation of SHBG appears to be important both for regulating clearance of the protein from the blood and the 0-linked glycosylation effects the action of SHBG on target cells (**Figure 1**) [19, 20].

SHBG contains a calcium-binding site in the N-terminal LG domain that may stabilize dimer formation [12]. Crystallographic studies demonstrate a zinc-binding

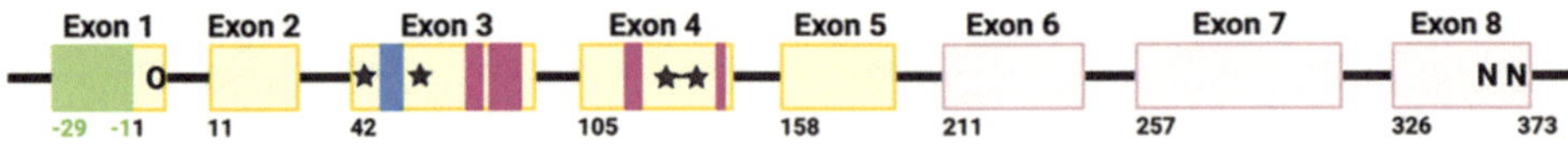

Figure 1.
SHBG gene structure. The SHBG gene is comprised of 8 exons encoding a mature protein of 373 amino acids with two laminin G-like (LG) domains. A 29 amino acid secretion signal sequence is encoded in exon 1 (green). Exons 2–5 (yellow) encode the N-terminal LG domain and exons 6–8 encode the C-terminal LG domain. Amino acids 42, 65, and 128–134 (stars) contribute to steroid binding. The regions that interact in SHBG dimer formation (magenta) are encoded by exons 3 and 4 (amino acids 72–77, 84–93, 119–126, 154–155). A region that has been shown to be required for SHBG to bind to cell surface receptors (blue) is encoded in exon 3 (amino acids 48–57). SHBG is O-glycosylated on Thr7 (O) and N-glycosylated on Asn351 and Asn367 (N). The amino acid encoded at the beginning of each exon is designated by the black numbers under each exon. This figure is based on figures in [6, 7]. Created in BioRender. Roberts, K. (2023) BioRender.com/d52k183.

site positioned close to the entrance to the steroid-binding site that reduces the affinity of SHBG for estrogens [21]. It follows that the high zinc concentrations in male reproductive tissues, such as the prostate and epididymis, may cause a shift towards an increased specificity of SHBG for androgens in these tissues.

3. SHBG gene expression patterns: Of mice and men

One of the differences between human and murine SHBG biology is the primary site of gene expression, protein synthesis, and secretion. In humans, SHBG is expressed in the liver and secreted into the bloodstream [22, 23]. In the rat, SHBG is expressed in the testis, principally in Sertoli cells, and secreted into the lumen of the seminiferous tubule [24, 25]. SHBG is also expressed in the testis of mice but at lower levels than that found in the rat [11].

Transgenic mice created using the rat SHBG gene, including 1.5 kb of upstream regulatory region, expressed the rat SHBG in a manner analogous to that in the rat, with high levels of expression in Sertoli cells but no expression in the liver or other tissues [26]. Some of the transgenic lines created had defects in spermatogenesis that were similar to that seen in testosterone deficient rats [27]. Transgenic mice created with a human SHBG transgene, with a similar length of regulatory region, expressed SHBG in the liver and kidneys but not in the testis [28]. The difference in tissue-specific expression between rat and human SHBG is attributed to a USF-1/USF-2 binding site in the proximal regulatory region of the human SHBG gene that is absent in the mouse and rat orthologs (**Figure 2**) [30]. When this regulatory element is removed from the human gene construct and used to create a transgenic mouse, the SHBG gene is transcribed in Sertoli cells, and its expression is stimulated by FSH, similar to that seen for endogenous mouse ABP [30].

Although the primary site of human SHBG production is the liver, low levels of immunoreactive SHBG have been detected in the human testis [31]. The testicular form of human SHBG is expressed in germ cells from a distal promoter, approximately 1.9 kb upstream of the transcription start site (**Figure 2**) [8]. Expression from this regulatory domain produces a transcript encoding an alternate exon 1. Although alternatively spliced forms of the transcript were described, the primary transcript appears to contain exons 2–8 [32]. The germ cell form of SHBG appears to be the product of translation that initiates from the codon for Met30 in exon 2 [32]. This alternative human SHBG transcript also accumulates in the germ cells of transgenic mice harboring the human SHBG transgene containing the upstream alternative exon 1 and upstream regulatory region [33]. Treatment of human and SHBG transgenic mouse sperm samples with N-glycosidase F demonstrated that the germ cell SHBG is N-glycosylated [32, 33]. Expression of the germ cell form of SHBG has been demonstrated in the GC2 mouse germ cell line where it appears to be controlled by SPZ1, a transcription factor highly expressed in germ cells, and CREB/CREM transcription factor family members (**Figure 2**) [34]. The germ cell SHBG appears to accumulate between the outer acrosomal membrane and the plasma membrane, and it is detected at all stages of spermatid development [33]. The germ cell isoform of SHBG is predicted to be without a signal polypeptide, consistent with its accumulation in germ cell cytoplasm [35]. Whether its role in the sperm is one of steroid retention or some other function is unknown.

It has been observed that proinflammatory cytokines can suppress the expression of SHBG in the human liver, and that the levels of SHBG in the bloodstream are inversely correlated with both Body Mass Index (BMI) and the fat content of the liver [29]. In overweight individuals, low serum levels of SHBG serve as an indicator of

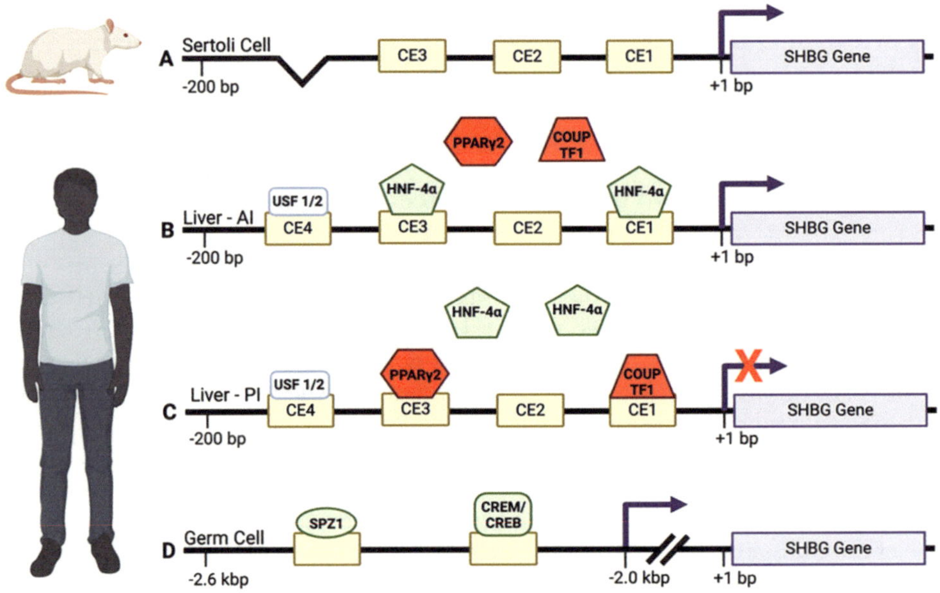

Figure 2.
Transcriptional control of SHBG expression. SHBG expression in murine Sertoli cells (A) and human liver (B,C) is regulated by cis-acting elements (CE) in the proximal promoter region of the gene. Liver-specific expression is determined by CE4, which is a binding site for transcription factors USF 1 and 2. The absence of this element in mice and rats results in Sertoli cell specific expression. Expression of SHBG in the human liver is dependent on physiological parameters that reflect disease states. Under pro-inflammatory (PI) conditions (C), HNF-4α is down regulated allowing PPARγ2 and COUP-TF1 to bind CE3 and CE1, respectively, and depress transcription of SHBG. Conversely, HNF-4α is upregulated under anti-inflammatory (AI) conditions and binds to CE1 and CE3, increasing expression of SHBG. Expression of SHBG in germ cells (D) is driven from an upstream regulatory region containing regulatory elements that bind SPZ1 and CREM/CREB. Transcription from this regulatory region encodes an alternate exon 1 and produces a transcript that initiates translation from a methionine codon in exon 2. This figure is based on figures in [7, 29]. Created in BioRender. Roberts, K. (2024) BioRender.com/p74b956.

metabolic syndrome and have been found to be predictive for cardiovascular disease and type 2 diabetes [36–39]. It is worth noting that SHBG levels may also be altered in other disease states [29, 40]. In women, low serum SHBG levels have been associated with polycystic ovary syndrome (PCOS) and with gestational diabetes [41, 42]. In fact, treatments that increase SHBG levels in patients with PCOS are correlated with positive treatment outcomes [43]. Therefore, SHBG levels may prove an important marker for patients at risk of PCOS and following SHBG levels a useful tool for monitoring treatment effectiveness [41, 43].

It is not clear whether SHBG is involved in the pathogenesis of these diseases and metabolic states or merely correlative, but SHBG levels are clearly influenced by inflammatory and metabolic processes. The transcription factor HNF-4α, a key driver of SHBG expression, is down-regulated by proinflammatory cytokines TNFα and IL1β, leading to a decrease in SHBG expression [44–47]. When the levels of HNF-4α are low, COUP-TF binds to the regulatory region and further reduces SHBG expression (**Figure 2**) [22]. Adiponectin, an anti-inflammatory protein with protective properties against metabolic syndrome, was shown to increase expression of SHBG by increasing the level of HNF-4α and lowering fatty acid levels by enhancing β -oxidation [48, 49]. The inhibitory effect of fatty acids on SHBG expression have been reproduced in a transgenic mouse expressing human SHBG [50]. Interestingly, the mono-unsaturated fatty acid oleate, elevates SHBG levels by down-regulating PPAR-α, a transcription factor that suppresses SHBG expression (**Figure 2**) [51].

In addition to its primary expression in the human liver and murine testis, SHBG has been shown to be expressed at low levels, and with many different splice variant forms, in many different tissues and cells [6, 25, 52, 53]. Taken together, the complex expression patterns of the SHBG/ABP gene suggest roles in processes beyond sex steroid binding and implicate this protein in many additional pathways.

4. SHBG binding and function

Historically, the predominant view on SHBG function in the circulation is, along with other binding proteins such as albumin, the binding of sex steroids and consequent effect on free hormone concentration. A number of different studies have demonstrated the high affinity binding of SHBG to testosterone and DHT, along with a lesser affinity for estradiol [54–56]. Some studies have also shown allosteric binding of steroids to SHBG [57, 58]. In men, the concentration of SHBG in serum ranges from 19 to 70 nM, a level sufficient to bind approximately 70% of the testosterone in serum (9–32 nM) and thereby influence the concentration of free testosterone [59–61].

While SHBG can bind the majority of testosterone in the blood and may have an influence on androgen regulation of target tissues, it is less likely that this is the case in the testis, where testosterone levels are very high compared to serum. Studies conducted by Jarrow and Zirkin measured intratesticular testosterone levels in human testicular aspirates and found them to range from thirty to over 100-fold higher than plasma levels [62, 63]. These studies also predicted that greater than 70% of this androgen is bioactive. The concentration of SHBG in the human testis averaged 8.5 nM, and thus, it would be predicted to have a minimal effect on the bioavailability of testosterone [62].

SHBG may, however, be important in situations where the levels of testosterone in the testis are low. Testosterone suppression in rats given testosterone and estradiol implants to suppress GnRH/LH production results in spermatogenic failure [64, 65]. In these animals, the testicular levels of testosterone, although dramatically reduced from normal levels, are still at least 2–3 times higher than normal serum levels. SHBG levels in the rat testis are seven times higher than in serum, and the concentration of SHBG is unaffected by falling testosterone levels [66, 67]. Roberts and Zirkin demonstrated that the concentration of rat SHBG relative to testosterone under these circumstances was sufficient to inhibit transcription from an androgen-responsive reporter construct, directly demonstrating an inhibitory effect of SHBG on androgen action [68].

The effect of rat SHBG on androgen action in the testis is therefore dependent on its concentration relative to testosterone. In mice, the SHBG level in the testis is much lower than that of the rat [11]. In transgenic mice expressing the human SHBG gene primarily in the liver, there is no effect on spermatogenesis [28]. But transgenic mice expressing the rat SHBG gene at high levels in Sertoli cells show a pronounced inhibition of spermatogenesis that is consistent with the decreased levels of bioavailable testosterone in these animals [69–71]. Microarray analysis of testis tissue in these same transgenic mice shows that gene expression is altered by the reduced levels of bioavailable testosterone [72]. The level of testosterone falls below the normal concentration of SHBG in the testis of men receiving a hormonal contraceptive regimen, suggesting the possibility that SHBG binding of testosterone contributes to the contraceptive effect [73].

The role of circulating SHBG in sequestering sex steroid hormones is also important in females. In cases of hirsutism and acne, if SHBG levels are low the condition is more likely to be caused by excess free androgen [74]. In women undergoing treatment for PCOS with the goal of obtaining a successful pregnancy, treatment that increases the level of SHBG and the resultant reduction in free androgen are strongly correlated to successful treatment [75].

5. Possible mediators of SHBG activity

The conclusion that SHBG acts by binding sex steroids and thereby regulating the bioavailable levels of these important hormones is consistent with, and likely influenced by, the well-accepted free hormone hypothesis [76]. But it is now clear that SHBG also interacts directly with proteins on the plasma membranes of specific cell types, and this may result in uptake of SHBG-bound sex steroids via endocytotic mechanisms and/or cell membrane receptor-mediated signaling [77, 78].

5.1 Receptor mediated uptake of SHBG

Uptake of SHBG has been demonstrated in several tissues and cell types, including the epididymis, uterus and uterine tube, brain, lymphocytes, and prostate and breast

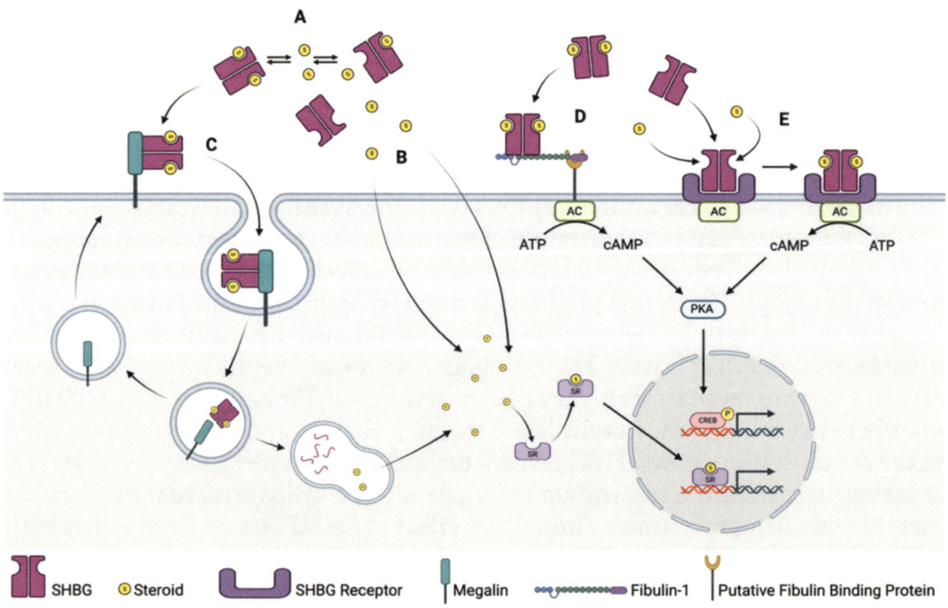

Figure 3.
SHBG mechanisms of action in mediating the physiological effects of sex steroid hormones (primarily androgens and estrogen). (A) Sex steroid hormones in blood and interstitial fluids are in equilibrium with SHBG creating a pool of free hormone, the concentration of which is dependent on concentration of SHBG. (B) Free steroid hormone can diffuse into target cells and bind the intracellular steroid hormone receptor (SR) and activate steroid-dependent gene transcription. (C) SHBG with steroid bound can bind to megalin and be taken up by receptor-mediated endocytosis. SHBG is degraded in the lysosome and free steroid hormone is released into the cell where it binds to the steroid hormone receptor. (D) SHBG can bind to fibulin-1 and, when estradiol is bound to the SHBG, activate adenylate cyclase via an unknown fibulin binding protein activating the cAMP-dependent second messenger signaling pathway. (E) SHBG without steroid bound can bind to a receptor on target cells. Subsequent binding of steroid hormone to receptor-bound SHBG results in the activation of adenylate cyclase and production of cAMP. This figure is based on figures in [40, 92, 93]. Created in BioRender. Roberts, K. (2024) BioRender.com/r81n129.

cancer cell lines [24, 79–85]. In the epididymis, rat SHBG was shown to increase the uptake of testosterone by epididymal epithelial cells over that achieved by free testosterone or DHT [83, 86]. In most tissues, the receptor(s) responsible for the mediated uptake of SHBG has not been established. However, strong experimental evidence supports a role for LDL Receptor-Related Protein 2 (LRP2), commonly known as megalin, in receptor mediated SHBG uptake in reproductive tissues [87].

Megalin, expressed at high levels in the kidney proximal tubule where it is important in protein uptake in proximal tubules, is also expressed in several reproductive tissues, including the epididymis, endometrium, mammary gland, and prostate cancer cells [88–90]. Megalin is known to bind a large number of different protein ligands, including SHBG [91]. In BN16 cells, a model cell line for assessing megalin-mediated uptake, megalin was shown to bind SHBG with high affinity and to internalize bound DHT, resulting in androgen-dependent gene expression (**Figure 3**) [87]. Moreover, male megalin-null mice have been shown to present with cryptorchidism, and female null mice with failure of vaginal opening, among other disorders of sexual development [87]. Cryptorchism can be reproduced by administration of anti-androgens during fetal development [94]. The male megalin-null mice also have reduced expression of several androgen-inducible genes (i.e., Tex12, Morc, Stk25, Ramp2) and an increased level of expression for androgen-repressed genes (i.e., Mpo and Igfbp5) [87]. Taken together, these studies provide evidence that sex steroid uptake via an SHBG-receptor binding and internalization pathway is important in sex steroid-dependent processes. Such a mechanism of sex steroid action may complement, and perhaps add specificity to, the free hormone mechanism of sex steroid action.

5.2 Cell surface receptors

SHBG has been shown to bind to specific receptors expressed on the plasma membrane of target cells [95–97]. This interaction has been most extensively characterized on breast cancer and prostate cancer cell lines [77, 98–100]. The SHBG receptor (R_{SHBG}) on the cell surface binds to unliganded SHBG [92]. The SHBG-R_{SHBG} complex is activated by subsequent binding of an appropriate androgen or estrogen [92, 101]. R_{SHBG} activation leads to a rapid increase in intracellular cAMP and activation of protein kinase A (**Figure 3**) [98, 99, 102–105]. Downstream effects of SHBG-R_{SHBG} binding in the prostate include increased prostate specific antigen expression and increased ALVA-41 prostate cancer cell growth [106, 107].

Studies by Nakhla et al. found that in human prostatic explants, estradiol, but not dihydrotestosterone, was active in generating cAMP via the SHBG-R_{SHBG} pathway [106]. There is evidence in lymphocytes that SHBG binds to a membrane-bound form of the estrogen receptor [79]. In the prostate this response appears not to be mediated by the estrogen receptor (ER), as evidenced by the lack of an effect of the estrogen agonist diethylstilbestrol, which does not bind to SHBG, and the inability of tamoxifen, an ER antagonist, to inhibit the response [106]. The response to estradiol via SHBG-R_{SHBG} was inhibited by anti-androgens, suggesting that the SHBG- R_{SHBG} pathway interacts with the androgen receptor signaling pathway in the human prostate.

The biological effects of SHBG signaling in breast cancer tissues and cells are well established. The SHBG-R_{SHBG} complex induces an increase in intracellular cAMP, a decrease in progesterone receptor expression, and induced apoptosis via the suppression of ERK signaling, culminating in an inhibition of breast tumor cell growth [21, 93, 98, 103, 108–113]. SHBG has been shown to bind to fibulin-1D and fibulin-2 in transgenic mice expressing the human SHBG gene and that this binding sequesters circulating SHBG in the endometrial stroma [114]. Fibulins comprise a family of secreted glycoproteins that localize to the basement membrane and interact with laminins and other proteins of the extracellular matrix. They are involved in cell adhesion, proliferation, migration, and differentiation, as well as influencing cancer progression [115, 116]. Marano et al. confirmed the interaction of fibulin-1 with SHBG and further demonstrated that fibulin-1 is required for the binding of SHBG to MCF-7 breast cancer cells [93]. Silencing fibulin expression in these cells alters estrogen-regulated gene expression, and importantly, these studies showed that silencing of fibulin expression results in more aggressive cell growth. In breast cancer tissues, positive fibulin expression correlated with a lower tumor grade [93]. Together, these results suggest that fibulin is involved in the receptor-mediated mechanism of SHBG action on these target cells (**Figure 3**).

The source of the SHBG that initializes R_{SHBG} signaling *in vivo* is unclear. It could be taken up from the plasma, where it is abundant in humans, or it may be synthesized in the tissues where signaling occurs. SHBG protein and mRNA have been demonstrated in human tissues as such as the prostate and breast, among others [52, 53, 117–119]. Although the concentration of SHBG changes between fetal development, puberty, and adult, it is not known if temporal changes in the concentration of plasma SHBG play a role in R_{SHBG} signaling [7]. Tissue-specific sites of expression, such as the prostate and breast, could control local SHBG concentrations, thereby regulating R_{SHBG} activation in an autocrine/paracrine manner. Alternatively, cell sensitivity to SHBG could be regulated by expression of the R_{SHBG}.

6. Novel mutants informing SHBG function

A few naturally occurring SHBG mutations have been described in the literature and each attest to the importance of SHBG to normal endocrine physiology. A single nucleotide change resulting in an Asp to Asn substitution at amino acid 327 results in an additional N-glycosylation site that extends the half-life of SHBG in circulation [120, 121]. The increased level of SHBG that results correlates with the preventive effect of SHBG on breast cancer and its inverse correlation to the incidence of type 2 diabetes [36, 122, 123]. A mutation resulting in a proline to leucine substitution at position 156 results in a decrease in affinity for testosterone and is correlated with a reduction in plasma testosterone levels in affected men [124]. Several other expressed single nucleotide variants in the SHBG gene have been biochemically characterized and shown to cause functional changes to the protein [125].

A striking example of the necessity for SHBG for normal physiology is described in a case report of a 27-year-old man homozygous for a missense mutation (G to A) that encodes a secretion defective SHBG variant resulting in undetectable SHBG in his blood [126]. As expected, plasma testosterone concentrations in the man were well below the normal range, yet his free testosterone levels were in the normal range. Clinical assessments indicated fatigue, overt muscle weakness, and low body weight, low libido, and other symptoms of hypoandrogenism. Semen analysis showed normal semen volume and sperm concentration and normal testicular volume. These finding suggest that intratesticular testosterone concentrations are sufficient to maintain testicular function and circulating testosterone is adequate for sex accessory gland function. Additionally, normal levels of LH indicated normal pituitary perception of testosterone availability. These finding suggest that plasma SHBG is not essential for male reproductive development and sperm production, but that SHBG supports the anabolic activities of androgens systemically. This implies that plasma SHBG is not required for normal male sexual development even if it results in a hypoandrogenic state in adulthood.

7. Summary and future directions

Over the past 40 years, substantial research has been conducted on SHBG, shedding light on its expression, mode of action, and its impact on human health. SHBG is known to bind androgens and estrogens with high affinity, effectively regulating the concentration of free steroid hormone in circulation. The protein can be internalized via receptor-mediated endocytosis, bound to megalin, and possibly other receptors, and this internalization has various biological effects. SHBG also binds to one or more cell surface receptors and activates second messenger systems that have profound effects on prostate, breast, and other cell types. We also know that SHBG levels inversely correlate with various medical conditions including metabolic syndrome, type 2 diabetes, and other inflammatory conditions. The regulatory region of the SHBG gene provides insight into these expression patterns, but it is unclear if decreased expression of SHBG contributes to the pathology of these conditions.

The human and murine orthologs of SHBG produce nearly identical proteins but do so from entirely different tissues. It is uncertain whether the actions of SHBG in humans and murine species are essentially the same or whether the difference in the site of synthesis leads to fundamentally different functions. Serum levels of human SHBG are much higher than those found in mice or rats, suggesting some difference in function. To better understand SHBG's function, it would be of great interest to create a humanized rat model carrying a human SHBG transgene expressed in the liver and a knockout of the endogenous testicular gene. Such a humanized model could be studied to determine the effect that the site of synthesis has on the function of SHBG. It may also prove useful for investigating the role of SHBG in obesity, metabolic syndrome, and other associated conditions.

Despite much research, the specific cell surface receptor for SHBG signaling remains unknown, although the most recent work suggests that the receptor may be fibulin-1. If this is the case, one might expect action of SHBG in the many different tissues that express fibulin-1. One might also expect a role for SHBG in development, where fibulin-1 has been shown to be important. Moreover, a definitive identification of a specific SHBG receptor would greatly increase our understanding of SHBG's function and provide a target for further investigation.

Finally, what is the function of the germ cell form of SHBG that has been found in human spermatids? Is it expressed in the germ cells of murine models as well? Its presence in germ cells suggests a role in sperm function and possibly in fertilization and/or early embryogenesis. A knockout mouse for SHBG has not been reported in the literature but would shed some light on these questions of essential SHBG function.

Conflict of interest

The authors declare no conflict of interest.

Author details

Kyle C. Schuppe and Kenneth P. Roberts*
Department of Translational Medicine and Physiology, Elson S. Floyd College of Medicine, Washington State University, Spokane, WA, USA

*Address all correspondence to: kenroberts@wsu.edu

References

[1] Gershagen S, Fernlund P, Lundwall A. A cDNA coding for human sex hormone binding globulin. Homology to vitamin K-dependent protein S. FEBS Letters. 1987;**220**(1):129-135. DOI: 10.1016/0014-5793(87)80890-6

[2] Hammond GL, Underhill DA, Smith CL, Goping IS, Harley MJ, Musto NA, et al. The cDNA-deduced primary structure of human sex hormone-binding globulin and location of its steroid-binding domain. FEBS Letters. 1987;**215**(1):100-104. DOI: 10.1016/0014-5793(87)80121-7

[3] Joseph DR, Hall SH, French FS. Identification of complementary DNA clones that encode rat androgen binding protein. Journal of Andrology. 1985;**6**(6):392-395. DOI: 10.1002/j.1939-4640.1985.tb03301.x

[4] Joseph DR, Hall SH, French FS. Rat androgen-binding protein: Evidence for identical subunits and amino acid sequence homology with human sex hormone-binding globulin. Proceedings of the National Academy of Sciences of the United States of America. 1987;**84**(2):339-343. DOI: 10.1073/pnas.84.2.339

[5] Que BG, Petra PH. Characterization of a cDNA coding for sex steroid-binding protein of human plasma. FEBS Letters. 1987;**219**(2):405-409. DOI: 10.1016/0014-5793(87)80261-2

[6] Nakhla AM, Hryb DJ, Rosner W, Romas NA, Xiang Z, Kahn SM. Human sex hormone-binding globulin gene expression- multiple promoters and complex alternative splicing. BMC Molecular Biology. 2009;**10**:37. DOI: 10.1186/1471-2199-10-37

[7] Hammond GL. Diverse roles for sex hormone-binding globulin in reproduction. Biology of Reproduction. 2011;**85**(3):431-441. DOI: 10.1095/biolreprod.111.092593

[8] Gershagen S, Lundwall A, Fernlund P. Characterization of the human sex hormone binding globulin (SHBG) gene and demonstration of two transcripts in both liver and testis. Nucleic Acids Research. 1989;**17**(22):9245-9258. DOI: 10.1093/nar/17.22.9245

[9] Hammond GL, Underhill DA, Rykse HM, Smith CL. The human sex hormone-binding globulin gene contains exons for androgen-binding protein and two other testicular messenger RNAs. Molecular Endocrinology. 1989;**3**(11):1869-1876. DOI: 10.1210/mend-3-11-1869

[10] Joseph DR, Hall SH, Conti M, French FS. The gene structure of rat androgen-binding protein: Identification of potential regulatory deoxyribonucleic acid elements of a follicle-stimulating hormone-regulated protein. Molecular Endocrinology. 1988;**2**(1):3-13. DOI: 10.1210/mend-2-1-3

[11] Wang YM, Sullivan PM, Petrusz P, Yarbrough W, Joseph DR. The androgen-binding protein gene is expressed in CD1 mouse testis. Molecular and Cellular Endocrinology. 1989;**63**(1-2):85-92. DOI: 10.1016/0303-7207(89)90084-1

[12] Bocchinfuso WP, Hammond GL. Steroid-binding and dimerization domains of human sex hormone-binding globulin partially overlap: Steroids and Ca^{2+} stabilize dimer formation. Biochemistry. 1994;**33**(35):10622-10629. DOI: 10.1021/bi00201a008

[13] Grishkovskaya I, Avvakumov GV, Sklenar G, Dales D, Hammond GL,

Muller YA. Crystal structure of human sex hormone-binding globulin: Steroid transport by a laminin G-like domain. The EMBO Journal. 2000;**19**(4):504-512. DOI: 10.1093/emboj/19.4.504

[14] Khan MS, Hryb DJ, Hashim GA, Romas NA, Rosner W. Delineation and synthesis of the membrane receptor-binding domain of sex hormone-binding globulin. The Journal of Biological Chemistry. 1990;**265**(30):18362-18365

[15] Avvakumov GV, Grishkovskaya I, Muller YA, Hammond GL. Resolution of the human sex hormone-binding globulin dimer interface and evidence for two steroid-binding sites per homodimer. The Journal of Biological Chemistry. 2001;**276**(37):34453-34457. DOI: 10.1074/jbc.M106274200

[16] Hildebrand C, Bocchinfuso WP, Dales D, Hammond GL. Resolution of the steroid-binding and dimerization domains of human sex hormone-binding globulin by expression in Escherichia coli. Biochemistry. 1995;**34**(10):3231-3238. DOI: 10.1021/bi00010a012

[17] Stirk HJ, Woolfson DN, Hutchinson EG, Thornton JM. Depicting topology and handedness in jellyroll structures. FEBS Letters. 1992;**308**(1):1-3. DOI: 10.1016/0014-5793(92)81036-l

[18] Walsh KA, Titani K, Takio K, Kumar S, Hayes R, Petra PH. Amino acid sequence of the sex steroid binding protein of human blood plasma. Biochemistry. 1986;**25**(23):7584-7590. DOI: 10.1021/bi00371a048

[19] Cousin P, Dechaud H, Grenot C, Lejeune H, Hammond GL, Pugeat M. Influence of glycosylation on the clearance of recombinant human sex hormone-binding globulin from rabbit blood. The Journal of Steroid Biochemistry and Molecular Biology. 1999;**70**(4-6):115-121. DOI: 10.1016/s0960-0760(99)00101-6

[20] Raineri M, Catalano MG, Hammond GL, Avvakumov GV, Frairia R, Fortunati N. O-glycosylation of human sex hormone-binding globulin is essential for inhibition of estradiol-induced MCF-7 breast cancer cell proliferation. Molecular and Cellular Endocrinology. 2002;**189**(1-2):135-143. DOI: 10.1016/s0303-7207(01)00725-0

[21] Avvakumov GV, Muller YA, Hammond GL. Steroid-binding specificity of human sex hormone-binding globulin is influenced by occupancy of a zinc-binding site. The Journal of Biological Chemistry. 2000;**275**(34):25920-25925. DOI: 10.1074/jbc.M004484200

[22] Janne M, Hammond GL. Hepatocyte nuclear factor-4 controls transcription from a TATA-less human sex hormone-binding globulin gene promoter. The Journal of Biological Chemistry. 1998;**273**(51):34105-34114. DOI: 10.1074/jbc.273.51.34105

[23] Pugeat M, Nader N, Hogeveen K, Raverot G, Dechaud H, Grenot C. Sex hormone-binding globulin gene expression in the liver: Drugs and the metabolic syndrome. Molecular and Cellular Endocrinology. 2010;**316**(1):53-59. DOI: 10.1016/j.mce.2009.09.020

[24] French FS, Ritzen EM. A high-affinity androgen-binding protein (ABP) in rat testis: Evidence for secretion into efferent duct fluid and absorption by epididymis. Endocrinology. 1973;**93**(1):88-95. DOI: 10.1210/endo-93-1-88

[25] Joseph DR. Structure, function, and regulation of androgen-binding protein/sex hormone-binding globulin. Vitamins and Hormones. 1994;**49**:197-280. DOI: 10.1016/s0083-6729(08)61148-6

[26] Reventos J, Sullivan PM, Joseph DR, Gordon JW. Tissue-specific expression of the rat androgen-binding protein/sex hormone-binding globulin gene in transgenic mice. Molecular and Cellular Endocrinology. 1993;**96**(1-2):69-73. DOI: 10.1016/0303-7207(93)90096-3

[27] Joseph DR, O'Brien DA, Sullivan PM, Becchis M, Tsuruta JK, Petrusz P. Overexpression of androgen-binding protein/sex hormone-binding globulin in male transgenic mice: Tissue distribution and phenotypic disorders. Biology of Reproduction. 1997;**56**(1):21-32. DOI: 10.1095/biolreprod56.1.21

[28] Janne M, Deol HK, Power SG, Yee SP, Hammond GL. Human sex hormone-binding globulin gene expression in transgenic mice. Molecular Endocrinology. 1998;**12**(1):123-136. DOI: 10.1210/mend.12.1.0050

[29] Simo R, Saez-Lopez C, Barbosa-Desongles A, Hernandez C, Selva DM. Novel insights in SHBG regulation and clinical implications. Trends in Endocrinology and Metabolism. 2015;**26**(7):376-383. DOI: 10.1016/j.tem.2015.05.001

[30] Selva DM, Hogeveen KN, Hammond GL. Repression of the human sex hormone-binding globulin gene in sertoli cells by upstream stimulatory transcription factors. The Journal of Biological Chemistry. 2005;**280**(6):4462-4468. DOI: 10.1074/jbc.M409616200

[31] Cheng CY, Musto NA, Gunsalus GL, Frick J, Bardin CW. There are two forms of androgen binding protein in human testes. Comparison of their protomeric variants with serum testosterone-estradiol binding globulin. The Journal of Biological Chemistry. 1985;**260**(9):5631-5640

[32] Selva DM, Bassas L, Munell F, Mata A, Tekpetey F, Lewis JG, et al. Human sperm sex hormone-binding globulin isoform: Characterization and measurement by time-resolved fluorescence immunoassay. The Journal of Clinical Endocrinology and Metabolism. 2005;**90**(11):6275-6282. DOI: 10.1210/jc.2005-1192

[33] Selva DM, Hogeveen KN, Seguchi K, Tekpetey F, Hammond GL. A human sex hormone-binding globulin isoform accumulates in the acrosome during spermatogenesis. The Journal of Biological Chemistry. 2002;**277**(47):45291-45298. DOI: 10.1074/jbc.M205903200

[34] Selva DM, Hammond GL. Human sex hormone-binding globulin is expressed in testicular germ cells and not in sertoli cells. Hormone and Metabolic Research. 2006;**38**(4):230-235. DOI: 10.1055/s-2006-925336

[35] Hammond GL, Bocchinfuso WP. Sex hormone-binding globulin: Gene organization and structure/function analyses. Hormone Research. 1996;**45**(3-5):197-201. DOI: 10.1159/000184787

[36] Ding EL, Song Y, Manson JE, Hunter DJ, Lee CC, Rifai N, et al. Sex hormone-binding globulin and risk of type 2 diabetes in women and men. The New England Journal of Medicine. 2009;**361**(12):1152-1163. DOI: 10.1056/NEJMoa0804381

[37] Laaksonen DE, Niskanen L, Punnonen K, Nyyssonen K, Tuomainen TP, Valkonen VP, et al. Testosterone and sex hormone-binding globulin predict the metabolic syndrome and diabetes in middle-aged men. Diabetes Care. 2004;**27**(5):1036-1041. DOI: 10.2337/diacare.27.5.1036

[38] Le TN, Nestler JE, Strauss JF 3rd, Wickham EP 3rd. Sex hormone-binding globulin and type 2 diabetes mellitus. Trends in Endocrinology and

Metabolism. 2012;**23**(1):32-40. DOI: 10.1016/j.tem.2011.09.005

[39] Sutton-Tyrrell K, Wildman RP, Matthews KA, Chae C, Lasley BL, Brockwell S, et al. Sex-hormone-binding globulin and the free androgen index are related to cardiovascular risk factors in multiethnic premenopausal and perimenopausal women enrolled in the study of women across the nation (SWAN). Circulation. 2005;**111**(10):1242-1249. DOI: 10.1161/01.CIR.0000157697.54255.CE

[40] Basualto-Alarcon C, Llanos P, Garcia-Rivas G, Troncoso MF, Lagos D, Barrientos G, et al. Classic and novel sex hormone binding globulin effects on the cardiovascular system in men. International Journal of Endocrinology. 2021;**2021**:5527973. DOI: 10.1155/2021/5527973

[41] Deswal R, Yadav A, Dang AS. Sex hormone binding globulin—An important biomarker for predicting PCOS risk: A systematic review and meta-analysis. Systems Biology in Reproductive Medicine. 2018;**64**(1):12-24. DOI: 10.1080/19396368.2017.1410591

[42] Faal S, Abedi P, Jahanfar S, Ndeke JM, Mohaghegh Z, Sharifipour F, et al. Sex hormone binding globulin for prediction of gestational diabetes mellitus in pre-conception and pregnancy: A systematic review. Diabetes Research and Clinical Practice. 2019;**152**:39-52. DOI: 10.1016/j.diabres.2019.04.028

[43] Goldstajn MS, Toljan K, Grgic F, Jurkovic I, Baldani DP. Sex hormone binding globulin (SHBG) as a marker of clinical disorders. Collegium Antropologicum. 2016;**40**(3):211-218

[44] Haffner SM, Katz MS, Stern MP, Dunn JF. Association of decreased sex hormone binding globulin and cardiovascular risk factors. Arteriosclerosis. 1989;**9**(1):136-143. DOI: 10.1161/01.atv.9.1.136

[45] Simo R, Barbosa-Desongles A, Hernandez C, Selva DM. IL1beta down-regulation of sex hormone-binding globulin production by decreasing HNF-4alpha via MEK-1/2 and JNK MAPK pathways. Molecular Endocrinology. 2012;**26**(11):1917-1927. DOI: 10.1210/me.2012-1152

[46] Simo R, Barbosa-Desongles A, Lecube A, Hernandez C, Selva DM. Potential role of tumor necrosis factor-alpha in downregulating sex hormone-binding globulin. Diabetes. 2012;**61**(2):372-382. DOI: 10.2337/db11-0727

[47] Simo R, Barbosa-Desongles A, Saez-Lopez C, Lecube A, Hernandez C, Selva DM. Molecular mechanism of TNFalpha-induced down-regulation of SHBG expression. Molecular Endocrinology. 2012;**26**(3):438-446. DOI: 10.1210/me.2011-1321

[48] Esfahani M, Movahedian A, Baranchi M, Goodarzi MT. Adiponectin: An adipokine with protective features against metabolic syndrome. Iranian Journal of Basic Medical Sciences. 2015;**18**(5):430-442

[49] Simo R, Saez-Lopez C, Lecube A, Hernandez C, Fort JM, Selva DM. Adiponectin upregulates SHBG production: Molecular mechanisms and potential implications. Endocrinology. 2014;**155**(8):2820-2830. DOI: 10.1210/en.2014-1072

[50] Selva DM, Hogeveen KN, Innis SM, Hammond GL. Monosaccharide-induced lipogenesis regulates the human hepatic sex hormone-binding globulin gene. The Journal of Clinical Investigation.

2007;**117**(12):3979-3987. DOI: 10.1172/JCI32249

[51] Saez-Lopez C, Soriguer F, Hernandez C, Rojo-Martinez G, Rubio-Martin E, Simo R, et al. Oleic acid increases hepatic sex hormone binding globulin production in men. Molecular Nutrition & Food Research. 2014;**58**(4):760-767. DOI: 10.1002/mnfr.201300304

[52] Hryb DJ, Nakhla AM, Kahn SM, St George J, Levy NC, Romas NA, et al. Sex hormone-binding globulin in the human prostate is locally synthesized and may act as an autocrine/paracrine effector. The Journal of Biological Chemistry. 2002;**277**(29):26618-26622. DOI: 10.1074/jbc.M202495200

[53] Moore KH, Bertram KA, Gomez RR, Styner MJ, Matej LA. Sex hormone binding globulin mRNA in human breast cancer: Detection in cell lines and tumor samples. The Journal of Steroid Biochemistry and Molecular Biology. 1996;**59**(3-4):297-304. DOI: 10.1016/s0960-0760(96)00121-5

[54] Petra PH, Griffin PR, Yates JR 3rd, Moore K, Zhang W. Complete enzymatic deglycosylation of native sex steroid-binding protein (SBP or SHBG) of human and rabbit plasma: Effect on the steroid-binding activity. Protein Science. 1992;**1**(7):902-909. DOI: 10.1002/pro.5560010708

[55] Pugeat MM, Dunn JF, Nisula BC. Transport of steroid hormones: Interaction of 70 drugs with testosterone-binding globulin and corticosteroid-binding globulin in human plasma. The Journal of Clinical Endocrinology and Metabolism. 1981;**53**(1):69-75. DOI: 10.1210/jcem-53-1-69

[56] Renoir JM, Mercier-Bodard C, Baulieu EE. Hormonal and immunological aspects of the phylogeny of sex steroid binding plasma protein. Proceedings of the National Academy of Sciences of the United States of America. 1980;**77**(8):4578-4582. DOI: 10.1073/pnas.77.8.4578

[57] Jasuja R, Spencer D, Jayaraj A, Peng L, Krishna M, Lawney B, et al. Estradiol induces allosteric coupling and partitioning of sex-hormone-binding globulin monomers among conformational states. iScience. 2021;**24**(6):102414. DOI: 10.1016/j.isci.2021.102414

[58] Zakharov MN, Bhasin S, Travison TG, Xue R, Ulloor J, Vasan RS, et al. A multi-step, dynamic allosteric model of testosterone's binding to sex hormone binding globulin. Molecular and Cellular Endocrinology. 2015;**399**:190-200. DOI: 10.1016/j.mce.2014.09.001

[59] Aribas E, Roeters van Lennep JE, De Rijke YB, Laven JSE, Ikram MA, Peeters RP, et al. Sex steroids and sex steroid-binding globulin levels amongst middle-aged and elderly men and women from general population. European Journal of Clinical Investigation. 2022;**52**(12):e13866. DOI: 10.1111/eci.13866

[60] Elmlinger MW, Kuhnel W, Ranke MB. Reference ranges for serum concentrations of lutropin (LH), follitropin (FSH), estradiol (E2), prolactin, progesterone, sex hormone-binding globulin (SHBG), dehydroepiandrosterone sulfate (DHEAS), cortisol and ferritin in neonates, children and young adults. Clinical Chemistry and Laboratory Medicine. 2002;**40**(11):1151-1160. DOI: 10.1515/CCLM.2002.202

[61] Travison TG, Vesper HW, Orwoll E, Wu F, Kaufman JM, Wang Y,

et al. Harmonized reference ranges for circulating testosterone levels in men of four cohort studies in the United States and Europe. The Journal of Clinical Endocrinology and Metabolism. 2017;**102**(4):1161-1173. DOI: 10.1210/jc.2016-2935

[62] Jarow JP, Chen H, Rosner TW, Trentacoste S, Zirkin BR. Assessment of the androgen environment within the human testis: Minimally invasive method to obtain intratesticular fluid. Journal of Andrology. 2001;**22**(4):640-645

[63] Jarow JP, Zirkin BR. The androgen microenvironment of the human testis and hormonal control of spermatogenesis. Annals of the New York Academy of Sciences. 2005;**1061**:208-220. DOI: 10.1196/annals.1336.023

[64] Awoniyi CA, Santulli R, Sprando RL, Ewing LL, Zirkin BR. Restoration of advanced spermatogenic cells in the experimentally regressed rat testis: Quantitative relationship to testosterone concentration within the testis. Endocrinology. 1989;**124**(3):1217-1223. DOI: 10.1210/endo-124-3-1217

[65] Zirkin BR, Santulli R, Awoniyi CA, Ewing LL. Maintenance of advanced spermatogenic cells in the adult rat testis: Quantitative relationship to testosterone concentration within the testis. Endocrinology. 1989;**124**(6):3043-3049. DOI: 10.1210/endo-124-6-3043

[66] Gunsalus GL, Musto NA, Bardin W. Immunoassay of androgen binding protein in blood: A new approach for study of the seminiferous tubule. Science. 1978;**200**(4337):65-66. DOI: 10.1126/science.635573

[67] Morris ID, Bardin CW, Musto NA, Thau R, Gunsalus GL. Androgen binding protein in serum, testis and epididymis following treatment with the leydig cell cytotoxic agent, ethylene dimethanesulphonate. International Journal of Andrology. 1988;**11**(2):153-163. DOI: 10.1111/j.1365-2605.1988.tb00991.x

[68] Roberts KP, Zirkin BR. Androgen binding protein inhibition of androgen-dependent transcription explains the high minimal testosterone concentration required to maintain spermatogenesis in the rat. Endocrine Journal. 1993;**1**:41-47

[69] Jeyaraj DA, Grossman G, Petrusz P. Dynamics of testicular germ cell apoptosis in normal mice and transgenic mice overexpressing rat androgen-binding protein. Reproductive Biology and Endocrinology. 2003;**1**:48. DOI: 10.1186/1477-7827-1-48

[70] Jeyaraj DA, Grossman G, Petrusz P. Altered bioavailability of testosterone in androgen-binding protein-transgenic mice. Steroids. 2005;**70**(10):704-714. DOI: 10.1016/j.steroids.2005.03.015

[71] Jeyaraj DA, Grossman G, Weaver C, Petrusz P. Dynamics of testicular germ cell proliferation in normal mice and transgenic mice overexpressing rat androgen-binding protein: A flow cytometric evaluation. Biology of Reproduction. 2002;**66**(4):877-885. DOI: 10.1095/biolreprod66.4.877

[72] Petrusz P, Jeyaraj DA, Grossman G. Microarray analysis of androgen-regulated gene expression in testis: The use of the androgen-binding protein (ABP)-transgenic mouse as a model. Reproductive Biology and Endocrinology. 2005;**3**:70. DOI: 10.1186/1477-7827-3-70

[73] Coviello AD, Bremner WJ, Matsumoto AM, Herbst KL, Amory JK, Anawalt BD, et al. Intratesticular testosterone concentrations comparable

with serum levels are not sufficient to maintain normal sperm production in men receiving a hormonal contraceptive regimen. Journal of Andrology. 2004;**25**(6):931-938. DOI: 10.1002/j.1939-4640.2004.tb03164.x

[74] Selby C. Sex hormone binding globulin: Origin, function and clinical significance. Annals of Clinical Biochemistry. 1990;**27**(Pt 6):532-541. DOI: 10.1177/000456329002700603

[75] Lin XF, Wu RR, Du J, Liao YC, Du Y, Ye Y, et al. Exploring the significance of sex hormone-binding globulin examination in the treament of women with polycystic ovarian syndrome (PCOS). Clinical and Experimental Obstetrics & Gynecology. 2015;**42**(3):315-320

[76] Mendel CM. The free hormone hypothesis: A physiologically based mathematical model. Endocrine Reviews. 1989;**10**(3):232-274. DOI: 10.1210/edrv-10-3-232

[77] Rosner W, Hryb DJ, Kahn SM, Nakhla AM, Romas NA. Interactions of sex hormone-binding globulin with target cells. Molecular and Cellular Endocrinology. 2010;**316**(1):79-85. DOI: 10.1016/j.mce.2009.08.009

[78] Willnow TE, Nykjaer A. Cellular uptake of steroid carrier proteins--mechanisms and implications. Molecular and Cellular Endocrinology. 2010;**316**(1):93-102. DOI: 10.1016/j.mce.2009.07.021

[79] Balogh A, Karpati E, Schneider AE, Hetey S, Szilagyi A, Juhasz K, et al. Sex hormone-binding globulin provides a novel entry pathway for estradiol and influences subsequent signaling in lymphocytes via membrane receptor. Scientific Reports. 2019;**9**(1):4. DOI: 10.1038/s41598-018-36882-3

[80] Caldwell JD, Shapiro RA, Jirikowski GF, Suleman F. Internalization of sex hormone-binding globulin into neurons and brain cells in vitro and in vivo. Neuroendocrinology. 2007;**86**(2):84-93. DOI: 10.1159/000107072

[81] Feldman M, Lea OA, Petrusz P, Tres LL, Kierszenbaum AL, French FS, et al. Purification from rat epididymis, characterization, and immunocytochemical localization. The Journal of Biological Chemistry. 1981;**256**(10):5170-5175

[82] Gerard A, Khanfri J, Gueant JL, Fremont S, Nicolas JP, Grignon G, et al. Electron microscope radioautographic evidence of in vivo androgen-binding protein internalization in the rat epididymis principal cells. Endocrinology. 1988;**122**(4):1297-1307. DOI: 10.1210/endo-122-4-1297

[83] Li H, Pham T, McWhinney BC, Ungerer JP, Pretorius CJ, Richard DJ, et al. Sex hormone binding globulin modifies testosterone action and metabolism in prostate cancer cells. International Journal of Endocrinology. 2016;**2016**:6437585. DOI: 10.1155/2016/6437585

[84] Noe G, Cheng YC, Dabike M, Croxatto HB. Tissue uptake of human sex hormone-binding globulin and its influence on ligand kinetics in the adult female rat. Biology of Reproduction. 1992;**47**(6):970-976. DOI: 10.1095/biolreprod47.6.970

[85] Porto CS, Gunsalus GL, Bardin CW, Phillips DM, Musto NA. Receptor-mediated endocytosis of an extracellular steroid-binding protein (TeBG) in MCF-7 human breast cancer cells. Endocrinology. 1991;**129**(1):436-445. DOI: 10.1210/endo-129-1-436

[86] Turner TT, Roddy MS. Intraluminal androgen binding protein alters

3H-androgen uptake by rat epididymal tubules in vitro. Biology of Reproduction. 1990;**43**(3):414-419. DOI: 10.1095/biolreprod43.3.414

[87] Hammes A, Andreassen TK, Spoelgen R, Raila J, Hubner N, Schulz H, et al. Role of endocytosis in cellular uptake of sex steroids. Cell. 2005;**122**(5):751-762. DOI: 10.1016/j.cell.2005.06.032

[88] Garcia JK, Krieger KD, Loitz C, Perez L, Richards ZA, Helou Y, et al. Regulation of prostate androgens by megalin and 25-hydroxyvitamin D status: Mechanism for high prostate androgens in African American men. Cancer Research Communications. 2023;**3**(3):371-382. DOI: 10.1158/2767-9764.CRC-22-0362

[89] Nielsen R, Christensen EI, Birn H. Megalin and cubilin in proximal tubule protein reabsorption: From experimental models to human disease. Kidney International. 2016;**89**(1):58-67. DOI: 10.1016/j.kint.2015.11.007

[90] Zheng G, Bachinsky DR, Stamenkovic I, Strickland DK, Brown D, Andres G, et al. Organ distribution in rats of two members of the low-density lipoprotein receptor gene family, gp330 and LRP/alpha 2MR, and the receptor-associated protein (RAP). The Journal of Histochemistry and Cytochemistry. 1994;**42**(4):531-542. DOI: 10.1177/42.4.7510321

[91] Marzolo MP, Farfan P. New insights into the roles of megalin/LRP2 and the regulation of its functional expression. Biological Research. 2011;**44**(1):89-105. DOI: 10.4067/S0716-97602011000100012

[92] Hryb DJ, Khan MS, Romas NA, Rosner W. The control of the interaction of sex hormone-binding globulin with its receptor by steroid hormones. The Journal of Biological Chemistry. 1990;**265**(11):6048-6054

[93] Marano F, Zunino V, Frairia R, Arvat E, Castellano I, Bosco O, et al. Fibulin-1 interacts with sex hormone binding globulin and is linked to less aggressive estrogen-dependent breast cancers. Life Sciences. 2018;**207**:372-380. DOI: 10.1016/j.lfs.2018.06.024

[94] Spencer JR, Torrado T, Sanchez RS, Vaughan ED Jr, Imperato-McGinley J. Effects of flutamide and finasteride on rat testicular descent. Endocrinology. 1991;**129**(2):741-748. DOI: 10.1210/endo-129-2-741

[95] Felden F, Leheup B, Fremont S, Bouguerne R, Egloff M, Nicolas JP, et al. The plasma membrane of epididymal epithelial cells has a specific receptor which binds to androgen-binding protein and sex steroid-binding protein. The Journal of Steroid Biochemistry and Molecular Biology. 1992;**42**(3-4):279-285. DOI: 10.1016/0960-0760(92)90130-b

[96] Fortunati N, Becchis M, Fissore F, Berta L, Catalano MG, Orsello M, et al. The hepatic receptor for sex steroid-binding protein: Study on a non-malignant cell line (Chang liver). Journal of Molecular Endocrinology. 1993;**11**(3):257-264. DOI: 10.1677/jme.0.0110257

[97] Frairia R, Fortunati N, Berta L, Fazzari A, Fissore F, Gaidano G. Sex steroid binding protein (SBP) receptors in estrogen sensitive tissues. The Journal of Steroid Biochemistry and Molecular Biology. 1991;**40**(4-6):805-812. DOI: 10.1016/0960-0760(91)90306-p

[98] Fissore F, Fortunati N, Comba A, Fazzari A, Gaidano G, Berta L, et al. The receptor-mediated action of sex steroid binding protein (SBP, SHBG): Accumulation of cAMP in MCF-7 cells

under SBP and estradiol treatment. Steroids. 1994;**59**(11):661-667. DOI: 10.1016/0039-128x(94)90023-x

[99] Nakhla AM, Khan MS, Rosner W. Biologically active steroids activate receptor-bound human sex hormone-binding globulin to cause LNCaP cells to accumulate adenosine 3′,5′-monophosphate. The Journal of Clinical Endocrinology and Metabolism. 1990;**71**(2):398-404. DOI: 10.1210/jcem-71-2-398

[100] Porto CS, Musto NA, Bardin CW, Gunsalus GL. Binding of an extracellular steroid-binding globulin to membranes and soluble receptors from human breast cancer cells (MCF-7 cells). Endocrinology. 1992;**130**(5):2931-2936. DOI: 10.1210/endo.130.5.1315262

[101] Kahn SM, Hryb DJ, Nakhla AM, Romas NA, Rosner W. Sex hormone-binding globulin is synthesized in target cells. The Journal of Endocrinology. 2002;**175**(1):113-120. DOI: 10.1677/joe.0.1750113

[102] Fortunati N, Fissore F, Fazzari A, Becchis M, Comba A, Catalano MG, et al. Sex steroid binding protein exerts a negative control on estradiol action in MCF-7 cells (human breast cancer) through cyclic adenosine 3′,5′-monophosphate and protein kinase A. Endocrinology. 1996;**137**(2):686-692. DOI: 10.1210/endo.137.2.8593818

[103] Fortunati N, Fissore F, Fazzari A, Piovano F, Catalano MG, Becchis M, et al. Estradiol induction of cAMP in breast cancer cells is mediated by foetal calf serum (FCS) and sex hormone-binding globulin (SHBG). The Journal of Steroid Biochemistry and Molecular Biology. 1999;**70**(1-3):73-80. DOI: 10.1016/s0960-0760(99)00092-8

[104] Nakhla AM, Ding VD, Khan MS, Romas NA, Rhodes L, Smith RG, et al. 5 alpha-Androstan-3 alpha,17 beta-diol is a hormone: Stimulation of cAMP accumulation in human and dog prostate. The Journal of Clinical Endocrinology and Metabolism. 1995;**80**(7):2259-2262. DOI: 10.1210/jcem.80.7.7541803

[105] Porto CS, Lazari MF, Abreu LC, Bardin CW, Gunsalus GL. Receptors for androgen-binding proteins: Internalization and intracellular signalling. The Journal of Steroid Biochemistry and Molecular Biology. 1995;**53**(1-6):561-565. DOI: 10.1016/0960-0760(95)00111-c

[106] Nakhla AM, Romas NA, Rosner W. Estradiol activates the prostate androgen receptor and prostate-specific antigen secretion through the intermediacy of sex hormone-binding globulin. The Journal of Biological Chemistry. 1997;**272**(11):6838-6841. DOI: 10.1074/jbc.272.11.6838

[107] Nakhla AM, Rosner W. Stimulation of prostate cancer growth by androgens and estrogens through the intermediacy of sex hormone-binding globulin. Endocrinology. 1996;**137**(10):4126-4129. DOI: 10.1210/endo.137.10.8828467

[108] Catalano MG, Frairia R, Boccuzzi G, Fortunati N. Sex hormone-binding globulin antagonizes the anti-apoptotic effect of estradiol in breast cancer cells. Molecular and Cellular Endocrinology. 2005;**230**(1-2):31-37. DOI: 10.1016/j.mce.2004.11.005

[109] Fazzari A, Catalano MG, Comba A, Becchis M, Raineri M, Frairia R, et al. The control of progesterone receptor expression in MCF-7 breast cancer cells: Effects of estradiol and sex hormone-binding globulin (SHBG). Molecular and Cellular Endocrinology. 2001;**172**(1-2):31-36. DOI: 10.1016/s0303-7207(00)00397-x

[110] Fortunati N, Becchis M, Catalano MG, Comba A, Ferrera P, Raineri M, et al. Sex hormone-binding globulin, its membrane receptor, and breast cancer: A new approach to the modulation of estradiol action in neoplastic cells. The Journal of Steroid Biochemistry and Molecular Biology. 1999;**69**(1-6):473-479. DOI: 10.1016/s0960-0760(99)00068-0

[111] Fortunati N, Fissore F, Fazzari A, Berta L, Benedusi-Pagliano E, Frairia R. Biological relevance of the interaction between sex steroid binding protein and its specific receptor of MCF-7 cells: Effect on the estradiol-induced cell proliferation. The Journal of Steroid Biochemistry and Molecular Biology. 1993;**45**(5):435-444. DOI: 10.1016/0960-0760(93)90012-l

[112] Fortunati N, Raineri M, Cignetti A, Hammond GL, Frairia R. Control of the membrane sex hormone-binding globulin-receptor (SHBG-R) in MCF-7 cells: Effect of locally produced SHBG. Steroids. 1998;**63**(5-6):282-284. DOI: 10.1016/s0039-128x(98)00021-x

[113] Nakhla AM, Leonard J, Hryb DJ, Rosner W. Sex hormone-binding globulin receptor signal transduction proceeds via a G protein. Steroids. 1999;**64**(3):213-216. DOI: 10.1016/s0039-128x(98)00084-1

[114] Ng KM, Catalano MG, Pinos T, Selva DM, Avvakumov GV, Munell F, et al. Evidence that fibulin family members contribute to the steroid-dependent extravascular sequestration of sex hormone-binding globulin. The Journal of Biological Chemistry. 2006;**281**(23):15853-15861. DOI: 10.1074/jbc.M512370200

[115] de Vega S, Iwamoto T, Yamada Y. Fibulins: multiple roles in matrix structures and tissue functions. Cellular and Molecular Life Sciences. 2009;**66**(11-12):1890-1902. DOI: 10.1007/s00018-009-8632-6

[116] Mahajan D, Kancharla S, Kolli P, Sharma AK, Singh S, Kumar S, et al. Role of Fibulins in embryonic stage development and their involvement in various diseases. Biomolecules. 2021;**11**:5. DOI: 10.3390/biom11050685

[117] Murayama Y, Hammond GL, Sugihara K. The SHBG gene and Hormone dependence of breast cancer: A novel mechanism of hormone dependence of MCF-7 human breast cancer cells based upon SHBG. Breast Cancer. 1999;**6**(4):338-343. DOI: 10.1007/BF02966450

[118] Sinnecker G, Hiort O, Kwan PW, DeLellis RA. Immunohistochemical localization of sex hormone-binding globulin in normal and neoplastic breast tissue. Hormone and Metabolic Research. 1990;**22**(1):47-50. DOI: 10.1055/s-2007-1004847

[119] Sinnecker G, Hiort O, Mitze M, Donn F, Neumann S. Immunohistochemical detection of a sex hormone binding globulin like antigen in tissue sections of normal human prostate, benign prostatic hypertrophy and normal human endometrium. Steroids. 1988;**52**(4):335-336. DOI: 10.1016/0039-128x(88)90134-1

[120] Cousin P, Dechaud H, Grenot C, Lejeune H, Pugeat M. Human variant sex hormone-binding globulin (SHBG) with an additional carbohydrate chain has a reduced clearance rate in rabbit. The Journal of Clinical Endocrinology and Metabolism. 1998;**83**(1):235-240. DOI: 10.1210/jcem.83.1.4515

[121] Power SG, Bocchinfuso WP, Pallesen M, Warmels-Rodenhiser S, Van Baelen H, Hammond GL. Molecular

analyses of a human sex hormone-binding globulin variant: Evidence for an additional carbohydrate chain. The Journal of Clinical Endocrinology and Metabolism. 1992;**75**(4):1066-1070. DOI: 10.1210/jcem.75.4.1400872

[122] Costantino L, Catalano MG, Frairia R, Carmazzi CM, Barbero M, Coluccia C, et al. Molecular mechanisms of the D327N SHBG protective role on breast cancer development after estrogen exposure. Breast Cancer Research and Treatment. 2009;**114**(3):449-456. DOI: 10.1007/s10549-008-0031-4

[123] Key T, Appleby P, Barnes I, Reeves G, Endogenous H, Collaborative BC, et al. Endogenous sex hormones and breast cancer in postmenopausal women: Reanalysis of nine prospective studies. Journal of the National Cancer Institute. 2002;**94**(8):606-616. DOI: 10.1093/jnci/94.8.606

[124] Ohlsson C, Wallaschofski H, Lunetta KL, Stolk L, Perry JR, Koster A, et al. Genetic determinants of serum testosterone concentrations in men. PLoS Genetics. 2011;**7**(10):e1002313. DOI: 10.1371/journal.pgen.1002313

[125] Wu TS, Hammond GL. Naturally occurring mutants inform SHBG structure and function. Molecular Endocrinology. 2014;**28**(7):1026-1038. DOI: 10.1210/me.2014-1058

[126] Vos MJ, Mijnhout GS, Rondeel JM, Baron W, Groeneveld PH. Sex hormone binding globulin deficiency due to a homozygous missense mutation. The Journal of Clinical Endocrinology and Metabolism. 2014;**99**(9):E1798-E1802. DOI: 10.1210/jc.2014-2055

Chapter 3

Sex Steroid Hormone Dynamics in Reproduction in Sheep

Sadat Salifu, Joshua Salifu Wuntimah Mogre, Frederick Yeboah Obese and Stephen A. Osei

Abstract

The endocrine regulation of mammalian reproductive function is fundamentally governed by the intricate interplay of the sex steroid hormones of the hypothalamic-pituitary-gonadal axis, oestrogens, progestogens and androgens. These hormones are critical in initiating sexual maturation and maintaining reproductive competence throughout an organism's reproductive life. Ovine models have proven invaluable in elucidating the complexities of sex steroid action in livestock reproduction, with broader implications for our understanding of human reproductive physiology. The exponential growth in our understanding of sex steroids and related reproductive hormones due to improved detection methods of these hormones and production of analogues has significantly improved our capacity to manipulate oestrous cycle events and to exert greater control over reproductive processes. However, several aspects of sex steroid function remain elusive. Notably, the precise nature of neuroendocrine signals that trigger the positive feedback action of estrogen (primarily oestradiol in ovine) in the hypothalamic-pituitary axis remains incompletely characterized. This review synthesizes current knowledge on sex steroid function in reproduction in ovine reproduction, highlighting both advances and persisting knowledge gaps.

Keywords: progesterone, estrogen, testosterone, steroidogenesis, oestrous, assisted reproductive technologies

1. Introduction

Sex steroid hormones are a class of hormones that play a crucial role in the development and regulation of reproductive function in mammals [1]. The principal steroid hormones involved in reproduction are the androgens (mainly testosterone), oestrogens (oestradiol, oestrone in sheep) and progestogens (progesterone). These hormones are primarily produced in the gonads (testes in the male and ovaries in the females), although small amounts are produced in the adrenal glands. These sex steroids share a similar biosynthetic pathway, originating from the precursor cholesterol [2], but the ultimate products produced depend on the availability of particular metabolizing enzymes available in the cell [3]. Sex steroids exert their effects through genomic and non-genomic mechanisms [4], influencing various physiological processes beyond reproduction, including metabolism, bone density and cognitive function [5]. Sheep have been extensively used as an animal model for studying reproductive endocrinology due to their similarity with other livestock species and even humans [6–8]. Key aspects of sex steroid function include the development of secondary sexual characteristics, oestrous cycle regulation, pregnancy maintenance, foetal development and puberty onset. Testosterone is the principal male androgen which regulates male sexual behavior [9, 10] and is required in high concentrations to support the development of spermatozoa in the Sertoli cells [11]. The development of precise means of measuring steroid hormones has made detailed monitoring of sex steroid hormones possible and provided insights into the workings of the oestrous cycle, enabling the development of various oestrous synchronization protocols for manipulating the oestrous cycle for enhanced production of livestock [12–15].

2. Sheep as a model for reproductive research

Obvious ethical considerations bar the use of human subjects for most scientific experimentation involving manipulations that would be considered harmful to the subjects [16, 17]. Sheep, as a translational model, have made an outstanding contribution to our understanding of many areas of biomedical research, including neurological [18] cardiovascular [19], immune system physiology and reproductive research [20–22]. Several advantages are associated with using the ovine model compared to rodents or cows. Sheep are less expensive to use, docile and easier to handle compared to other large animal models such as cows which are more expensive and have a nearly two-year gestation period. Compared to rodent models, sheep also have a relatively long lifespan, enabling the study of critical processes over a longer period. Anatomically, their body size is closer to humans, and they share several physiological similarities with humans, which makes them amenable to intermittent and regular hormonal profiling compared to rodents [18].

The sheep model enables the examination of placental vascular development, placental nutrient exchange and the collection of repetitive foetal and maternal blood samples in order to understand maternal-foetal interactions due to functional similarities between human and sheep placentae [23]. Although sheep and humans have different gestation lengths (175 and 280 days, respectively), major developmental milestones during gestation are achieved at approximately similar stages, permitting comparisons between sheep and humans [24].

3. Synthesis of sex steroid hormones

3.1 Pathways of steroidogenesis

Steroidogenesis is the biosynthesis of steroid hormones from cholesterol. All steroid hormones share a similar biosynthetic pathway (**Figure 1**). The cholesterol precursor for steroid hormone synthesis is produced by the liver and is available for conversion via a series of steps involving several enzymes and systematic cleaving of cholesterol sidechains. The translocation of cholesterol to the inner mitochondrion by StAR protein for conversion to pregnenolone is the rate-limiting step in steroid biosynthesis [25, 26]. Steroidogenic acute regulatory (StAR) protein facilitates the entry of cholesterol into the inner mitochondria where the enzymatic cleaving of cholesterol begins. Steroid synthesis involves two types of enzymes: cytochrome P450 (CYP), which

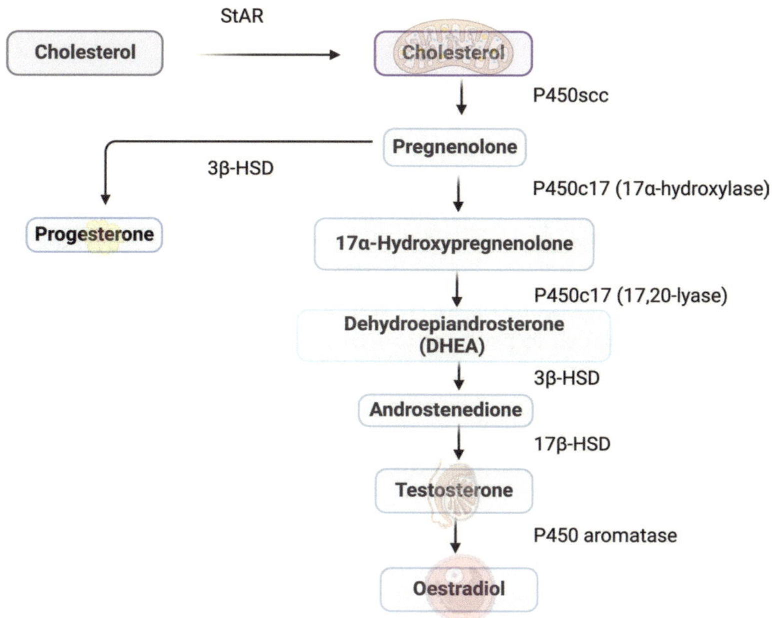

Figure 1.
The steroidogenic pathway of sex steroid hormones. (Image produced with Biorender.com).

are haeme-containing proteins that primarily catalyze hydroxylation reactions, and hydroxysteroid dehydrogenases (HSD), which play a role in oxidation and reduction reactions [27]. The mitochondria of the steroid-producing tissues such as the adrenals and gonads are inhabited by numerous steroidogenic enzymes such as the cholesterol side cleavage enzymes P450scc (cholesterol side-chain cleavage enzyme) [2].

3.2 Gene expressions and enzymes associated with sex steroid synthesis

Steroid hormone synthesis is governed by the Cytochrome P450 oxidative enzymes (**Table 1**).

Gene	Enzyme	Role
Cyp11a1	P450scc	Catalyzes the conversion of cholesterol to pregnenolone, the first committed step in steroid biosynthesis.
STAR	StAR	StAR facilitates the movement of cholesterol from the outer mitochondrial membrane to the inner mitochondrial membrane, a key step for steroidogenesis.
CYP19a1	P450aro/aromatase	converts androgens to oestrogens.
Cyp17a1	17α-Hydroxylase/17,20-Lyase	Converts pregnenolone to progesterone and catalyzes the formation of androgens (DHEA).
Hsd3b1	3β-Hydroxysteroid dehydrogenase type 1	Converts pregnenolone to progesterone and DHEA to androstenedione.

Table 1.
Genes and associated enzymes involved in sex steroid steroidogenesis.

3.3 Mechanism of action of sex steroid hormones

Like most steroid hormones, sex steroids exert their effects by diffusing freely across the cell membrane due to its lipophilic nature, and directly binding to intracellular receptors in the cell [25, 27]. They subsequently bind to specific intracellular receptors: estrogen binds to estrogen receptors ERα and ERβ; testosterone binds to androgen receptor (AR) and progesterone binds to progesterone receptor (PR). The hormone-receptor complex undergoes conformational changes, traverses the nuclear membrane and binds to specific spots on the DNA called hormone receptor elements (HREs). The complex alters gene expression by switching off or on genes, which ultimately influences the cell to produce more or less of certain proteins required to create the desired physiological effect.

4. Triggers and feedback mechanisms of steroid hormones in sheep

The hypothalamus-pituitary-gonadal axis regulates the complex interactions between the central nervous system and the reproductive axis, which involves a tightly controlled secretion of neurotransmitters and hormones. The control system of these hormones is called the positive and negative feedback mechanisms (**Figure 2**). Negative feedback, by far, is the principal mechanism by which sex steroid hormones are regulated [28]. Sex steroid hormones released from the gonads (ovaries and testes), under stimulation by gonadotropins, interact with the sites where their production is initiated, namely the hypothalamus and the pituitary gland to limit further production of the hormone, by downregulating the production of intermediary hormones, gonadotropin-releasing hormone (GnRH) and consequently, follicle-stimulating hormone (FSH) and luteinizing hormone (LH), in the negative feedback process [29]. When sex steroids such as progesterone rise (during the luteal phase or pregnancy), it suppresses the hypothalamic release of GnRH secretion, which

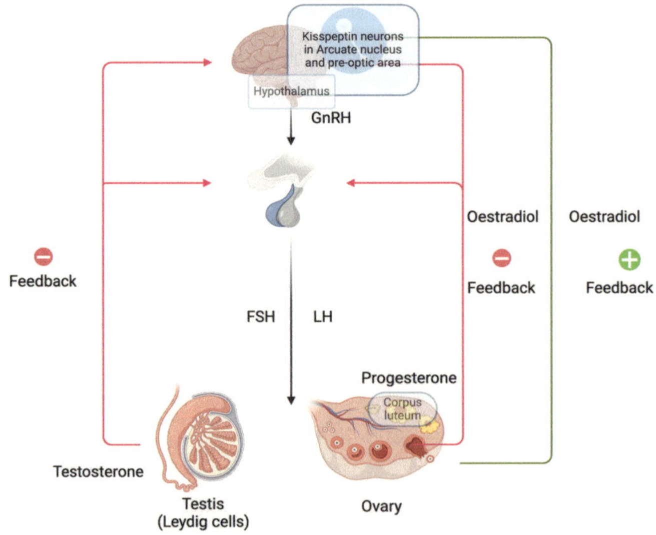

Figure 2.
The positive and negative feedback regulation of the hypothalamic-pituitary-gonadal axis steroid hormones. (Image produced with Biorender.com).

consequently lowers the production of LH and FSH. This decrease in gonadotropins leads to reduced stimulation of the gonads, thereby inhibiting follicular growth and lowering the production of oestradiol. Once progesterone levels decline, due to luteolysis of the corpus luteum or end of pregnancy, the negative feedback effect is removed, leading to secretion of GnRH, FSH and LH and resumption of follicular growth.

The less common positive feedback mechanism is observed in the stimulation of the GnRH surge centre in the neuroendocrine system during ovulation where a threshold concentration of oestradiol from the dominant follicle stimulates the kisspeptin neurons [30] in the arcuate and pre-optic area of the hypothalamus to stimulate a GnRH surge, which triggers the pre-ovulatory LH surge.

During puberty in lambs, the positive feedback effect of oestradiol is again observed as the initial high sensitivity of GnRH neurons gradually reduces, permitting higher doses of oestradiol until a threshold amount of oestradiol stimulates the surge centre to trigger the pre-ovulatory LH surge [29].

5. Roles of sex steroids in reproductive processes

Sex steroids are fundamental to the reproductive process and govern the interactions between the central nervous system (CNS) and the gonads.

5.1 Functions in male reproductive system

Testosterone is the main male androgen. Testosterone is primarily secreted by the Leydig cells under stimulation by LH in the testes [1]. Testosterone is responsible for the maturation of sperm in the Sertoli cells and promotion of growth, differentiation and function of accessory reproductive organs [31]. Testosterone is also responsible for male sexual behavior, including aggressive behavior [9, 32].

In sheep, testosterone synthesis and secretion begin in utero, once sexual differentiation occurs after day 35 [29, 33], where testosterone is produced by the male foetus to aid in the development and differentiation of the male reproductive organs. There is evidence from *in vitro* studies that the testes and mesonephros (embryological kidney) have the competence to produce testosterone before sexual differentiation as all the enzymes required for testosterone synthesis are present [33].

At the neonatal stage, the capacity for testosterone production is initially low, but there is an increase in testosterone which continues to support the development of the testes. In male lambs, the sustained increase in LH secretion from about 8 weeks of age signals the initiation of neuroendocrine puberty [34]. Average testosterone secretion in the male increases in an age-dependent fashion. From 3 months to about 17 months of age, there is an age-related increase in testosterone level in the ram lamb from 1.83 ng/ml to 13.28 ng/ml [35, 36] to support the maturation of the testes and the beginning of spermatogenesis.

5.2 Functions in female reproductive system

In sheep, ovarian follicular development is continuous, regardless of the stage of the oestrous cycle [37]. Within each oestrous cycle, three or four follicular waves occur where follicles are recruited and start to grow and produce oestradiol, with some follicles becoming atretic [38–41]. In the follicular phase of the oestrus cycle, oestradiol is produced by the granulosa cells of the ovulatory antral follicles, which can number as many as four in sheep. At threshold amounts, the negative feedback of oestradiol switches to positive feedback for continuous production of GnRH and LH leading to ovulation.

6. Stages of the reproductive process

6.1 Sex steroid hormone changes during puberty in the female

Female animals have their full complement of follicles at birth [42, 43], but their development is in an arrested state, and only basal levels of oestradiol are produced, which is not sufficient initially to trigger positive feedback. The initiation of puberty in the female sheep requires the pulsatile secretion of GnRH from the GnRH surge centre to generate a sufficient (threshold) amount of estrogen leading to the LH surge. The positive feedback mechanism is initially inhibited by a highly sensitive negative feedback mechanism where low concentrations of estrogen inhibit GnRH secretion [35]. With approaching puberty, the sensitivity of the GnRH surge centre in the ewe lamb decreases gradually, permitting larger quantities of oestradiol to be produced, which eventually reaches the threshold required to stimulate the GnRH surge centre leading to the LH surge and ovulation [44, 45].

In sheep, the first oestrus may be missed ("quiet oestrus") due to the absence of progesterone priming required to stimulate sexual behavior in the ewe lamb [46]. The corpus luteum formed after this initial ovulation however supplies the progesterone priming needed for exhibition of sexual behavior in subsequent ovulations [47, 48].

6.2 Hormonal dynamics of the sheep oestrous cycle

Oestrous cycles represent repeated opportunities for the female animal to become pregnant [29]. Oestrous cycles are continuous year-round in equatorial regions of Earth where variation in daylight hours is very little year-round [49]. Temperate sheep however experience oestrous cyclicity during the breeding season and undergo seasonal anoestrus, a period of reproductive quiescence [33] during which breeding activity ceases for several months (usually spring and summer); they are therefore referred to as seasonally polyestrous [49].

The reference point for the start of the sheep oestrous cycle is the observation of oestrus, when the female permits mating by the ram [49, 50]. The event of oestrus therefore marks the starting point of the oestrous cycle, and the cycle is defined as the period between two successive matings/oestruses. The starting point of the sheep oestrous cycle is one of several important differences between the ovine oestrous cycle and the oestrous cycle in human females. The reference point for the 28-day menstrual cycle of women begins from the time the uterine lining is shed (menstruation) for about 5 days in the absence of conception [51, 52]. In contrast to the length of the menstrual cycle, sheep have an average oestrous cycle length of 17 days [42], divided into four distinct phases: proestrus, oestrus, metestrus and dioestrus. The proestrus and oestrus periods mark the follicular phase of the oestrous cycle, where oestradiol is produced by the growing follicles under stimulation by FSH, while the metestrus and dioestrus mark the luteal phase, where progesterone is produced by the corpus luteum under stimulation by LH. In humans, sexual receptivity is not restricted to the oestrus period [51].

The onset of oestrus is closely preceded by an increase in oestradiol levels, which are secreted by the granulosa of the antral follicle [40]. Oestradiol rises in response to increasing growth and differentiation of theca and granulosa cells which acquire the competence to produce oestradiol [50]. This rise in oestradiol is crucial as it not only promotes the expression of female sexual behavior but also enhances the receptivity of males. Additionally, oestradiol plays a vital role in preparing the tubular genital tract and uterus for the potential implantation of an embryo.

The elevation of oestradiol levels initiates a positive feedback loop when it reaches a critical threshold, ultimately resulting in a surge of luteinizing hormone (LH). This LH surge is a pivotal event that triggers ovulation. Subsequently, following ovulation, the corpus luteum is formed and begins to secrete progesterone, a process regulated by LH. Progesterone secretion typically persists for approximately 12 days; however, if fertilization does not occur, this secretion is curtailed due to the influence of prostaglandin F2α (PGF2α). The regression of the corpus luteum removes the inhibitory effects on follicular development, allowing for a renewed phase of follicular growth driven by FSH. Ovulation occurs midway (14 days) through the cycle in women, and the corpus luteum is shortly formed and starts to secrete progesterone and some estrogen, which promotes endometrial growth. Towards the end of the cycle, the corpus luteum undergoes luteolysis if the woman does not become pregnant, and progesterone undergoes a sharp decline. With the sudden decline in progesterone, hormonal support for the endometrial lining is removed, resulting in the shedding of the ovarian lining (menstruation), marking the beginning of a new cycle [51].

6.3 The role of sex steroids in pregnancy and parturition

Progesterone is the dominant sex steroid during pregnancy as it is critical to pregnancy establishment, development of the early conceptus [53–55] and pregnancy maintenance via inhibition of oxytocin to keep a quiescent uterus throughout pregnancy [56, 57]. Progesterone also facilitates gene expression for nutrient transporters at the pre-implantation stage [58]. Following implantation, progesterone contributes to the elongation of the conceptus and elaboration of interferon tau (IFNT), a protein responsible for the maternal recognition of pregnancy [59, 60]. Maternal recognition of pregnancy inhibits the regression of the corpus luteum which continues to produce progesterone to support pregnancy [61, 62]. The corpus luteum in sheep produces progesterone for the first 30 days of pregnancy until the substantial placental contribution adds to it [63, 64]. As in sheep, the corpus luteum continues to produce progesterone until the placenta takes over. Hormonal administration is necessary in humans when progesterone production from the corpus luteum is insufficient in the first trimester of pregnancy [65]. However, luteoplacental shift occurs from 8 to 9 weeks of pregnancy, and the corpus luteum only contributes minimally in late pregnancy [65].

Gestation lasts for approximately 150 days in sheep. It is believed that space limitations for the foetus initiate the events of parturition by activating the hypothalamic-pituitary adrenal axis to produce corticotropin-releasing hormone (CRH), adrenocorticotrophic hormone (ACTH) and eventually cortisol by the foetal adrenal glands. The foetal corticoids activate the enzymes 17α-hydroxylase, 17–20 desmolase and aromatase which convert progesterone to estrogen. This conversion explains the precipitous drop in progesterone which removes the restraining influence of progesterone (progesterone block) on myometrial activity [51, 66], culminating in contractions and expulsion of the lamb.

7. Measurement of sex steroid hormones

Hormone assays have seen wide application in reproductive physiology research [13, 14, 67] and techniques have been developed to detect them in various body fluids, including blood [47], urine [68] and milk [69]. The accurate measurement of sex steroids is an invaluable research and diagnostic tool in veterinary medicine [70]. Sex steroid measurements have been invaluable in elucidating the workings of the reproductive system and can be used as a management tool for pregnancy diagnosis [71, 72], anovulation diagnosis (ovulation failure) or early pregnancy loss.

Steroid hormones have been detectable with a high level of accuracy with the advent of tools like radioimmunoassays (RIAs) [73] and enzyme-linked immunosorbent assays (ELISAs) [74, 75].

8. Sex steroids in reproductive dysfunction

Proper functioning of the reproductive axis requires the synthesis and secretion of adequate concentrations of hormones in a precisely timed manner. Where there are inadequate amounts, or poorly timed secretion of hormones, this has been linked to various pathological conditions. Exposure to sex steroid mimics and premature/prolonged exposure to some sex steroids have been associated with pathology.

Prenatal exposure to excess androgens, as well as glucocorticoids, and endocrine-disrupting chemicals (EDCs) with steroidogenic activity can disrupt the development of the foetus, resulting in adult disease [76]. This is because improper exposure to steroids or steroid mimics during critical periods of development can disrupt the typical course of organ system development. The metabolic system is especially vulnerable to the negative effects of this prenatal steroid excess. Prenatal exposure to excess native steroids or EDCs with steroidogenic activity, such as bisphenol A, can result in numerous cardiometabolic problems after birth [77]. These problems include insulin resistance, increased adiposity, changes in both adipocyte size and distribution and hypertension.

In female sheep, premature chronic exposure to oestrogenic compounds from subterranean clover (*Trifolium subterraneum*) is linked to delayed onset of puberty [78, 79].

Polycystic ovarian syndrome (PCOS) has long been known as a complicated reproductive and metabolic disease [80], characterized by chronic anovulation, hyperandrogenism, insulin resistance and polycystic ovaries [81, 82]. Ovine models have been critical to the study of polycystic ovarian syndrome (PCOS) in human females. Prenatal exposure to testosterone has been implicated in PCOS, as exposing female sheep fetuses to excess androgens during pregnancy predisposes them to metabolic and reproductive disorders in adulthood, akin to PCOS in humans [24, 76, 83]. Using Finnish Landrace X Dorset Horn sheep, Clarke et al. [84] exposed sheep to excess testosterone at different windows during pregnancy and showed that the critical time of exposure that resulted in masculinization of the foetus was day 40 to day 50. The extensive studies [85–87] using manipulation of prenatal testosterone in ewes to create a PCOS phenotype that provides a ready model for studying the progression of PCOS in women would not be ethical in human studies, making sheep a valuable subject in PCOS research [24].

9. Therapeutic and pharmacologic uses of sex steroids

The control of oestrus and ovulation has led to significant advances in sheep production such as synchronized lambing, higher fertility and fecundity, induction of out-of-season breeding and advancement of puberty in lambs [60]. This has been largely achieved using vaginal sponges or controlled internal drug release devices (CIDRs) impregnated with synthetic progestogens like flourogestone acetate (FGA) [88] and medroxyprogesterone acetate (MDA) [89] that mimic the luteal phase of oestrus cycle by inhibiting GnRH and gonadotropin hormones, paving the way for synchronized follicular development and ovulation once the progesterone is removed.

10. Conclusion

Sex steroid hormones are integral to sheep reproduction, influencing everything from sexual development and behavior to the intricacies of the oestrous cycle and pregnancy maintenance. The three primary sex steroids—oestrogens, progestogens and androgens—are primarily produced in the gonads, with sheep serving as valuable models for understanding their roles. Advancements in hormone measurement techniques, particularly RIAs and ELISAs, have been instrumental in understanding these hormones and their functions. These insights have led to significant advancements in sheep production, including oestrous synchronization, out-of-season breeding and improved fertility. Manipulation of the oestrous cycle, largely through the use of synthetic progestogens, has revolutionized sheep farming practices. However, several aspects of sex steroid function, especially the triggers for positive estrogen feedback, remain areas of ongoing research. Further research into the intricacies of these hormones promises even greater advancements in sheep breeding and management practices.

Conflict of interest

The authors declare no conflict of interest.

Author details

Sadat Salifu[1*], Joshua Salifu Wuntimah Mogre[1], Frederick Yeboah Obese[2] and Stephen A. Osei[3]

1 Council for Scientific and Industrial Research—Animal Research Institute, Tamale, Ghana

2 Department of Animal Science, School of Agriculture and Consumer Sciences, University of Ghana, Accra, Ghana

3 Department of Animal Science, Kwame Nkrumah University for Science and Technology, Kumasi, Ghana

*Address all correspondence to: ssalifuari@gmail.com

References

[1] Tremblay JJ. Molecular regulation of steroidogenesis in endocrine Leydig cells. Steroids. 2015;**103**:3-10. DOI: 10.1016/j.steroids.2015.08.001

[2] Papadopoulos V, Miller WL. Role of mitochondria in steroidogenesis. Best Practice & Research. Clinical Endocrinology & Metabolism. 2012;**26**(6):771-790. DOI: 10.1016/j.beem.2012.05.002

[3] Miller WL, Auchus RJ. The molecular biology, biochemistry, and physiology of human steroidogenesis and its disorders. Endocrine Reviews. 2011;**32**(1):81-151. DOI: 10.1210/er.2010-0013

[4] Simoncini T, Genazzani AR. Non-genomic actions of sex steroid hormones. European Journal of Endocrinology. 2003;**148**(3):281-292. DOI: 10.1530/eje.0.1480281

[5] Delchev S, Georgieva K, Delchev S, Georgieva K. Cellular and molecular mechanisms of the effects of sex hormones on the nervous system. In: Sex Hormones in Neurodegenerative Processes and Diseases. London, UK: IntechOpen; 2017. DOI: 10.5772/intechopen.71140

[6] Barry JS, Anthony RV. The pregnant sheep as a model for human pregnancy. Theriogenology. 2008;**69**(1):55-67. DOI: 10.1016/j.theriogenology.2007.09.021

[7] Montenegro L et al. The contribution of the sheep and the goat model to the study of ovarian ageing. Biology. 2023;**12**(2):270. DOI: 10.3390/biology12020270

[8] Martin GB. Frontiers in sheep reproduction - making use of natural responses to environmental challenges to manage productivity. Animal Reproduction. 2022;**19**(4):e20220088. DOI: 10.1590/1984-3143-ar2022-0088

[9] Preston BT, Stevenson IR, Lincoln GA, Monfort SL, Pilkington JG, Wilson K. Testes size, testosterone production and reproductive behaviour in a natural mammalian mating system. The Journal of Animal Ecology. 2012;**81**(1):296-305. DOI: 10.1111/j.1365-2656.2011.01907.x

[10] Pelletier F, Bauman J, Festa-Bianchet M. Fecal testosterone in bighorn sheep (*Ovis canadensis*): Behavioural and endocrine correlates. Canadian Journal of Zoology. 2003;**81**(10):1678-1684. DOI: 10.1139/z03-156

[11] Zhao W, Adjei M, Zhang Z, Yuan Z, Cisang Z, Song T. The role of GnRH in Tibetan male sheep and goat reproduction. Reproduction in Domestic Animals. 2023;**58**(9):1179-1187. DOI: 10.1111/rda.14432

[12] Salifu S. The Reproductive Performance of Djallonke Sheep in the Northern Region of Ghana, Master of Philosophy. Kumasi, Ghana: Kwame Nkrumah University for Science and Technology, Kumasi; 2014

[13] Tuah AK et al. Effects of levels of cocoa pod husk and NaOH-treated corn cob on the reproductive performance of Djallonké sheep. Tropical Agriculture, Trinidad and Tobago. 1999;**76**(2):131-135

[14] Salifu S, Avornyo F, Panyan E, Hagan B. Influence of season of lambing on postpartum interval to ovarian activity in Djallonke ewes. International Journal of Livestock Research. 2018;**8**(5):50. DOI: 10.5455/ijlr.20180224114616

[15] Santos-Jimenez Z, Martinez-Herrero C, Encinas T, Martinez-Ros P, Gonzalez-Bulnes A. Comparative efficiency of oestrus synchronization in sheep with progesterone/eCG and progesterone/GnRH during breeding and non-breeding season. Reproduction in Domestic Animals. 2020;**55**(7):882-884. DOI: 10.1111/rda.13698

[16] Komesaroff P, Dodds S, McNeill P, Skene L, Thomson C. Human Research Ethics Handbook: Commentary on the National Statement on Ethical Conduct in Research Involving Humans. Tasmania, Australia: University of Tasmania, report [Online]; 2002. Available from: https://figshare.utas.edu.au/articles/report/Human_Research_Ethics_Handbook_Commentary_on_the_National_Statement_on_Ethical_Conduct_in_Research_Involving_Humans/23166938/1 [Accessed: October 10, 2024]

[17] Mathur R, Swaminathan S. National ethical guidelines for biomedical & health research involving human participants, 2017: A commentary. The Indian Journal of Medical Research. 2018;**148**(3):279. DOI: 10.4103/0971-5916.245303

[18] Murray SJ, Mitchell NL. The translational benefits of sheep as large animal models of human neurological disorders. Frontiers in Veterinary Science. 2022;**9**:831838. DOI: 10.3389/fvets.2022.831838

[19] Camacho P, Fan H, Liu Z, He J-Q. Large mammalian animal models of heart disease. Journal of Cardiovascular Development and Disease. 2016;**3**(4):30. DOI: 10.3390/jcdd3040030

[20] Paping A et al. A sustainable translational sheep model for planned cesarean delivery of contraction-free ewes. Reproductive Sciences. 2024;**31**(3):791-802. DOI: 10.1007/s43032-023-01365-y

[21] Atik A et al. Long-term pulmonary effects of intrauterine exposure to endotoxin following preterm birth in sheep. Reproductive Sciences. 2012;**19**(12):1352-1364. DOI: 10.1177/1933719112450327

[22] Brown LD et al. Fetal sex does not impact placental blood flow or placental amino acid transfer in late gestation pregnant sheep with or without placental insufficiency. Reproductive Sciences. 2022;**29**(6):1776-1789. DOI: 10.1007/s43032-021-00750-9

[23] Banstola A, Reynolds JNJ. The sheep as a large animal model for the investigation and treatment of human disorders. Biology. 2022;**11**(9):1251. DOI: 10.3390/biology11091251

[24] Padmanabhan V, Veiga-Lopez A. Sheep models of polycystic ovary syndrome phenotype. Molecular and Cellular Endocrinology. 2013;**373**(1-2):8-20. DOI: 10.1016/j.mce.2012.10.005

[25] Miller WL, Bose HS. Early steps in steroidogenesis: Intracellular cholesterol trafficking. Journal of Lipid Research. 2011;**52**(12):2111-2135. DOI: 10.1194/jlr.R016675

[26] Miller WL. Steroidogenesis: Unanswered questions. Trends in Endocrinology and Metabolism. 2017;**28**(11):771-793. DOI: 10.1016/j.tem.2017.09.002

[27] Payne AH, Hales DB. Overview of steroidogenic enzymes in the pathway from cholesterol to active steroid hormones. Endocrine Reviews. 2004;**25**(6):947-970. DOI: 10.1210/er.2003-0030

[28] Herbison AE. A simple model of estrous cycle negative and positive feedback regulation of GnRH secretion. Frontiers in Neuroendocrinology.

2020;**57**:100837. DOI: 10.1016/j.yfrne.2020.100837

[29] Senger PL. Pathways to Pregnancy and Parturition. 2nd ed. Washington, USA: Current Conceptions Ltd; 2003

[30] Adachi S et al. Involvement of anteroventral periventricular Metastin/Kisspeptin neurons in estrogen positive feedback action on luteinizing hormone release in female rats. The Journal of Reproduction and Development. 2007;**53**(2):367-378. DOI: 10.1262/jrd.18146

[31] Freeman ER, Bloom DA, McGuire EJ. A brief history of testosterone. The Journal of Urology. 2001;**165**(2):371-373. DOI: 10.1097/00005392-200102000-00004

[32] Hull EM, Dominguez JM. Male sexual behavior. In: Knobil and Neill's Physiology of Reproduction. California, USA: Elsevier; 2015. pp. 2211-2285. DOI: 10.1016/B978-0-12-397175-3.00049-1

[33] Smith JT. The role of kisspeptin and gonadotropin inhibitory hormone in the seasonal regulation of reproduction in sheep. Domestic Animal Endocrinology. 2012;**43**(2):75-84. DOI: 10.1016/j.domaniend.2011.11.003

[34] Kosut SS, Wood RI, Herbosa-Encarnación C, Foster DL. Prenatal androgens time neuroendocrine puberty in the sheep: Effect of testosterone dose. Endocrinology. 1997;**138**(3):1072-1077. DOI: 10.1210/endo.138.3.4993

[35] Maksimović N et al. Development of sexual behaviour in ram lambs and its correlation to serum testosterone. Large Animal Review. 2021;**27**:31-34

[36] Maksimović N et al. Investigation of serum testosterone level, scrotal circumference, body mass, semen characteristics, and their correlations in developing MIS lambs. Turkish Journal of Veterinary and Animal Sciences. 2016;**40**:53-59. DOI: 10.3906/vet-1505-61

[37] Goodman RL, Inskeep EK. Control of the ovarian cycle of the sheep. In: Knobil and Neill's Physiology of Reproduction. California, USA: Elsevier; 2015. pp. 1259-1305. DOI: 10.1016/B978-0-12-397175-3.00027-2

[38] Ginther OJ, Kot K, Wiltbank MC. Associations between emergence of follicular waves and fluctuations in FSH concentrations during the estrous cycle in ewes. Theriogenology. 1995;**43**(3):689-703. DOI: 10.1016/0093-691X(94)00074-5

[39] Bartlewski PM, Baby TE, Giffin JL. Reproductive cycles in sheep. Animal Reproduction Science. 2011;**124**(3-4):259-268. DOI: 10.1016/j.anireprosci.2011.02.024

[40] Evans ACO. Ovarian follicle growth and consequences for fertility in sheep. Animal Reproduction Science. 2003;**78**(3-4):289-306. DOI: 10.1016/S0378-4320(03)00096-4

[41] Bartlewski PM, Beard AP, Cook SJ, Chandolia RK, Honaramooz A, Rawlings NC. Ovarian antral follicular dynamics and their relationships with endocrine variables throughout the oestrous cycle in breeds of sheep differing in prolificacy. Reproduction. 1999;**115**(1):111-124. DOI: 10.1530/jrf.0.1150111

[42] Picton HM. Activation of follicle development: The primordial follicle. Theriogenology. 2001;**55**(6):1193-1210. DOI: 10.1016/S0093-691X(01)00478-2

[43] Monniaux D et al. Follicular growth and ovarian dynamics in mammals.

Journal of Reproduction and Fertility. Supplement. 1997;**51**:3-23

[44] Valasi I, Chadio S, Fthenakis GC, Amiridis GS. Management of pre-pubertal small ruminants: Physiological basis and clinical approach. Animal Reproduction Science. 2012;**130**(3-4): 126-134. DOI: 10.1016/j.anireprosci. 2012.01.005

[45] Foster DL. Preovulatory gonadotropin surge system of prepubertal female sheep is exquisitely sensitive to the stimulatory feedback action of estradiol*. Endocrinology. 1984;**115**(3):1186-1189. DOI: 10.1210/ endo-115-3-1186

[46] Scaramuzzi RJ, Tillson SA, Thorneycroft IH, Caldwell BV. Action of exogenous progesterone and estrogen on behavioral estrus and luteinizing hormone levels in the ovariectomized ewe. Endocrinology. 1971;**88**(5):1184-1189. DOI: 10.1210/endo-88-5-1184

[47] Salifu S, Osei SA, Allegye-Cudjoe E, Avornyo FK. Assessing the age of puberty of Djallonke gimmers born in rainy or dry season using progesterone measurements [Online]. Livestock Research for Rural Development. 2018;**30**(12):1-9. Available from: http:// www.lrrd.org/lrrd30/12/ssali30205.html

[48] Robinson TJ. The necessity for progesterone with estrogen for the induction of recurrent estrus in the ovariectomized ewe. Endocrinology. 1954;**55**(4):403-408. DOI: 10.1210/ endo-55-4-403

[49] Jainudeen MR, Wahid H, Hafez ESE. Sheep and goats. In: Hafez ESE, Hafez B, editors. Reproduction in Farm Animals. 7th ed. Maryland, USA: Lippincott William and Wilkins; 2000. pp. 172-181

[50] Hafez ESE, Hafez B. Folliculogenesis, egg maturation, and ovulation. In: Reproduction in Farm Animals. 7th ed. Maryland, USA: Wiley-Blackwell; 2000. p. 185

[51] Senger PL. Pathways to Pregnancy & Parturition. 3rd ed. Redmond, OR: Current Conceptions; 2012

[52] Strauss JF, Williams CJ. Ovarian life cycle. In: Yen and Jaffe's Reproductive Endocrinology. Philadelphia, USA: Elsevier; 2019. pp. 167-205.e9. DOI: 10.1016/ B978-0-323-47912-7.00008-1

[53] Bairagi S, Grazul-Bilska AT, Borowicz PP, Reyaz A, Valkov V, Reynolds LP. Placental development during early pregnancy in sheep: Progesterone and estrogen receptor protein expression. Theriogenology. 2018;**114**:273-284. DOI: 10.1016/j. theriogenology.2018.04.002

[54] Reynolds LP et al. Placental development during early pregnancy in sheep: Estrogen and progesterone receptor messenger RNA expression in pregnancies derived from *in vivo*–produced and *in vitro*–produced embryos. Domestic Animal Endocrinology. 2015;**53**:60-69. DOI: 10.1016/j.domaniend.2015.05.003

[55] Wiltbank MC et al. Physiological and practical effects of progesterone on reproduction in dairy cattle. Animal. 2014;**8**:70-81. DOI: 10.1017/ S1751731114000585

[56] Sfakianaki AK, Norwitz ER. Mechanisms of progesterone action in inhibiting prematurity. The Journal of Maternal-Fetal & Neonatal Medicine. 2006;**19**(12):763-772. DOI: 10.1080/14767050600949829

[57] Shu-Rong Z, Bremme K, Eneroth P, Nordberg A. The regulation *in vitro* of placental release of human chorionic gonadotropin, placental lactogen, and

prolactin: Effects of an adrenergic beta-receptor agonist and antagonist. American Journal of Obstetrics and Gynecology. 1982;**143**(4):444-450. DOI: 10.1016/0002-9378(82)90088-6

[58] Halloran KM et al. Pre-implantation exogenous progesterone and pregnancy in sheep. II. Effects on fetal-placental development and nutrient transporters in late pregnancy. Journal of Animal Science and Biotechnology. 2021;**12**(1):46. DOI: 10.1186/s40104-021-00567-1

[59] Godkin JD, Bazer FW, Moffatt J, Sessions F, Roberts RM. Purification and properties of a major, low molecular weight protein released by the trophoblast of sheep blastocysts at day 13-21. Reproduction. 1982;**65**(1):141-150. DOI: 10.1530/jrf.0.0650141

[60] Gonzalez-Bulnes A, Menchaca A, Martin GB, Martinez-Ros P. Seventy years of progestagen treatments for management of the sheep oestrous cycle: Where we are and where we should go. Reproduction, Fertility, and Development. 2020;**32**(5):441-452. DOI: 10.1071/RD18477

[61] Ranilla MJ, Sulon J, Carro MD, Mantecón AR, Beckers JF. Plasmatic profiles of pregnancy-associated glycoprotein and progesterone levels during gestation in churra and merino sheep. Theriogenology. 1994;**42**(3):537-545. DOI: 10.1016/0093-691x(94)90691-b

[62] Hoskins EC et al. Pre-implantation exogenous progesterone and pregnancy in sheep: I. Polyamines, nutrient transport, and progestamedins. Journal of Animal Science and Biotechnology. 2021;**12**(1):39. DOI: 10.1186/s40104-021-00554-6

[63] Flint AP, Burton RD, Heap RB. Sources of progesterone during gestation in barbary sheep (*Ammotragus lervia*). The Journal of Endocrinology. 1983;**98**(2):283-288. DOI: 10.1677/joe.0.0980283

[64] Heap RB, Galil AK, Harrison FA, Jenkin G, Perry JS. Progesterone and oestrogen in pregnancy and parturition: Comparative aspects and hierarchical control. Ciba Foundation Symposium. 1977;**47**:127-157. DOI: 10.1002/9780470720295.ch7

[65] Duncan WC. The inadequate corpus luteum. Reproduction and Fertility. 2021;**2**(1):C1-C7. DOI: 10.1530/RAF-20-0044

[66] Zakar T, Hertelendy F. Progesterone withdrawal: Key to parturition. American Journal of Obstetrics and Gynecology. 2007;**196**(4):289-296. DOI: 10.1016/j.ajog.2006.09.005

[67] Obese FY, Dwumah K, Adjorlolo LK, Ayizanga RA. Effects of feed supplementation on growth, blood parameters and reproductive performance in Sanga and Friesian-Sanga cows grazing natural pasture. Tropical Animal Health and Production. 2018;**50**(8):1739-1746. DOI: 10.1007/s11250-018-1614-7

[68] Sugianto NA, Dehnhard M, Newman C, Macdonald DW, Buesching CD. A non-invasive method to assess the reproductive status of the European badger (*Meles meles*) from urinary sex-steroid metabolites. General and Comparative Endocrinology. 2021;**301**:113655. DOI: 10.1016/j.ygcen.2020.113655

[69] Shemesh M, Ayalon N, Mazor T. Early pregnancy diagnosis in the ewe, based on milk progesterone levels. Reproduction. 1979;**56**(1):301-304. DOI: 10.1530/jrf.0.0560301

[70] Obese FY, MacCarthy C, Osei-Amponsah R, Ayizanga RA, Damptey JK.

Blood metabolite profiles in cycling and non-cycling Friesien-Sanga cross-bred cows grazing natural pasture during the post-partum period. Reproduction in Domestic Animals. 2015;**50**(2):304-311. DOI: 10.1111/rda.12492

[71] Alexander B et al. Early pregnancy diagnosis by serum progesterone and ultrasound in sheep carrying somatic cell nuclear transfer-derived pregnancies. Reproduction in Domestic Animals. 2008;**43**(2):207-211. DOI: 10.1111/j.1439-0531.2007.00878.x

[72] Ganaie BA, Khan MZ, Islam R, Makhdoomi DM, Qureshi S, Wani GM. Evaluation of different techniques for pregnancy diagnosis in sheep. Small Ruminant Research. 2009;**85**(2-3):135-141. DOI: 10.1016/j.smallrumres.2009.09.003

[73] Goldsmith SJ. Radioimmunoassay: Review of basic principles. Seminars in Nuclear Medicine. 1975;**5**(2):125-152. DOI: 10.1016/S0001-2998(75)80028-6

[74] Hornbeck PV. Enzyme-linked immunosorbent assays. Current Protocols in Immunology. 2015;**110**(1):1-23. DOI: 10.1002/0471142735.im0201s110

[75] Hornbeck P. Enzyme-linked immunosorbent assays. Current Protocols in Immunology. 1992;**1**(1):1-22. DOI: 10.1002/0471142735.im0201s01

[76] Cardoso RC, Padmanabhan V. Prenatal steroids and metabolic dysfunction: Lessons from sheep. Annual Review of Animal Biosciences. 2019;7:337-360. DOI: 10.1146/annurev-animal-020518-115154

[77] Kandaraki E et al. Endocrine disruptors and polycystic ovary syndrome (PCOS): Elevated serum levels of bisphenol a in women with PCOS. The Journal of Clinical Endocrinology and Metabolism. 2011;**96**(3):E480-E484. DOI: 10.1210/jc.2010-1658

[78] Adams NR. Detection of the effects of phytoestrogens on sheep and cattle. Journal of Animal Science. 1995;**73**(5):1509-1515. DOI: 10.2527/1995.7351509x

[79] Foster DL, Ryan KD, Goodman RL, Legan SJ, Karsch FJ, Yellon SM. Delayed puberty in lambs chronically treated with oestradiol. Reproduction. 1986;**78**(1):111-117. DOI: 10.1530/jrf.0.0780111

[80] Stein IF, Leventhal ML. Amenorrhea associated with bilateral polycystic ovaries. American Journal of Obstetrics and Gynecology. 1935;**29**(2):181-191. DOI: 10.1016/S0002-9378(15)30642-6

[81] Ehrmann DA. Polycystic ovary syndrome. The New England Journal of Medicine. 2005;**352**(12):1223-1236. DOI: 10.1056/NEJMra041536

[82] The Rotterdam ESHRE/ASRM-sponsored PCOS consensus workshop group. Revised 2003 consensus on diagnostic criteria and long-term health risks related to polycystic ovary syndrome (PCOS). Human Reproduction. 2004;**19**(1):41-47. DOI: 10.1093/humrep/deh098

[83] Gurule S, Sustaita-Monroe J, Padmanabhan V, Cardoso R. Developmental programming of the neuroendocrine axis by steroid hormones: Insights from the sheep model of PCOS. Frontiers in Endocrinology. 2023;**14**:1096187. DOI: 10.3389/fendo.2023.1096187

[84] Clarke IJ, Scaramuzzi RJ, Short RV. Effects of testosterone implants in pregnant ewes on their female offspring. Journal of Embryology and Experimental Morphology. 1976;**36**(1):87-99

[85] Padmanabhan V, Sarma HN, Savabieasfahani M, Steckler TL, Veiga-Lopez A. Developmental reprogramming of reproductive and metabolic dysfunction in sheep: Native steroids vs. environmental steroid receptor modulators. International Journal of Andrology. 2010;**33**(2):394-404. DOI: 10.1111/j.1365-2605.2009.01024.x

[86] Short RV. Sexual differentiation of the brain of the sheep. In: Forest MG, Bertrand J, editors. Sexual Endocrinology of the Perinatal Period. Lyon, France: Inserm; 1974. pp. 121-142

[87] Clarke IJ, Scaramuzzi RJ, Short RV. Ovulation in prenatally androgenized ewes. The Journal of Endocrinology. 1977;**73**(2):385-389. DOI: 10.1677/joe.0.0730385

[88] Swelum AA-A, Alowaimer AN, Abouheif MA. Use of fluorogestone acetate sponges or controlled internal drug release for estrus synchronization in ewes: Effects of hormonal profiles and reproductive performance. Theriogenology. 2015;**84**(4):498-503. DOI: 10.1016/j.theriogenology.2015.03.018

[89] Garoussi MT, Mavadati O, Bahonar M, Ragh MJ. The effect of medroxyprogesterone acetate with or without eCG on conception rate of fat-tail ewes in out of breeding season. Tropical Animal Health and Production. 2020;**52**(4):1617-1622. DOI: 10.1007/s11250-019-02159-8

Section 2

Progestins

Chapter 4

Role of Progestins in Reproduction

Godspower Onyeso, Japheth David, Michael Egwu and Menizibeya Welcome

Abstract

Progestins are artificial derivatives of the naturally occurring steroid progesterone and include most if not all, aspects of reproductive physiology and medicine. The functions of progestins are established in regulating menstruation, sustaining pregnancy, and treating infertility. This chapter provides detailed insights into the development, mechanism of action, classification of progestins, and their diverse roles in reproduction, with a particular focus on their roles in menstruation, ovulation, pregnancy, birth control, endometriosis, hormonal replacement therapy (HRT), and assisted reproductive technology (ART). The main discoveries indicate that progestins effectively control menstrual cycles, prevent premature ovulation, and facilitate the early maintenance of pregnancy. In contraceptive applications, they successfully inhibit ovulation and alter endometrial receptivity to prevent pregnancy. In treating endometriosis, progestins induce atrophy of endometrial lesions, providing significant symptom relief. In hormone replacement therapy (HRT), the effects of estrogen are regulated to alleviate symptoms of menopause and reduce the risk of endometrial hyperplasia. For ART, progestins enhance the conditions for successful embryo transfer and improve fertility outcomes. The overall recommendation is to continue progestin research to optimize their use in reproductive health, improve treatment protocols, and enhance patient outcomes, as that will help enhance the field of reproductive medicine.

Keywords: progestins, reproductive health, contraception, hormone replacement therapy, assisted reproductive technology

1. Introduction

Progestins are the homologues of the naturally occurring progesterone hormone. Because of their activity in the process of reproduction, progestins have been used in clinical practice for a long time in menstrual abnormalities, contraception, and HRT, among the various conditions affecting female reproductive health [1, 2]. Besides the regulation of the menstrual cycle, they also feature in pregnancy, ovulation, and fertility enhancement and form a cornerstone for modern reproductive medicine. However, their great diversity and dissimilar biological effects face the challenge of decision-making on the best formulation for specific applications in reproductive health.

The problem that becomes the basis for the development of this chapter is that the action of progestins in the reproduction system is so complicated. Even though progestin is generally used in contraceptive techniques, its use has been utilised in methods for fertility enhancement and treatment of diseases like endometriosis and menopause; the exact manner in which the various roles of progestins in reproduction is not clear [3, 4]. This translates to a gap in the optimisation of progestin use for the care and outcomes in female patients and the improvement of reproductive health. Therefore, further elucidation of progestins' role in differing aspects of reproduction is needed to develop enhanced therapeutic protocols and improve patient outcomes.

The overall aim of this chapter is to elaborate on progestins and their structures and critically explain their role in reproductive health, especially their mechanism of action in menstruation, ovulation, pregnancy, contraception, endometriosis, hormone replacement therapy (HRT), and artificial reproductive technology (ART).

The chapter aims specifically to achieve the following objectives:

1. To understand and discuss progestins – definition, chemical structure, mechanisms of action, and classifications.

2. To determine progestins' roles in regulating menstruation, ovulation, pregnancy, and contraception.

3. To understand the roles of progestins in managing reproductive medicine, including but not limited to the treatment of endometriosis, hormone replacement therapy, and assisted reproductive technology.

2. Progestin and female reproductive health

2.1 Understanding progestins

2.1.1 Definition of progestins

Progestins are synthetic steroid hormones that are developed to mimic the functions of progesterone (P4; natural progestogen) and are used for reproductive health and contraceptive purposes [1]. The hormone is essential for maintaining the physiologic functions of female reproductive processes like ovulation and sustaining a pregnancy [1, 2]. Progestins, also called synthetic progestogen hormones, interact with the nuclear receptors in the endometrium. They regulate functions such as gland inhibition, decidualisation, and the movement of white blood cells. The impact of progestins is influenced by the amount administered, the duration of use, and whether oestrogen is present [5].

P4, on the other hand, is a steroid hormone with a 21-carbon skeleton. It is mainly produced by the ovaries, adrenal glands, and testes. It plays a role in the female reproductive cycle, particularly in ovulation, the transformation of the endometrium, and the support of pregnancy [1, 6]. It is derived from cholesterol, which is converted into pregnenolone by the enzyme cytochrome P450scc and then transformed into P4 by the enzyme 3β-hydroxysteroid dehydrogenase (3-β-HSD) (See **Figure 1**) [1].

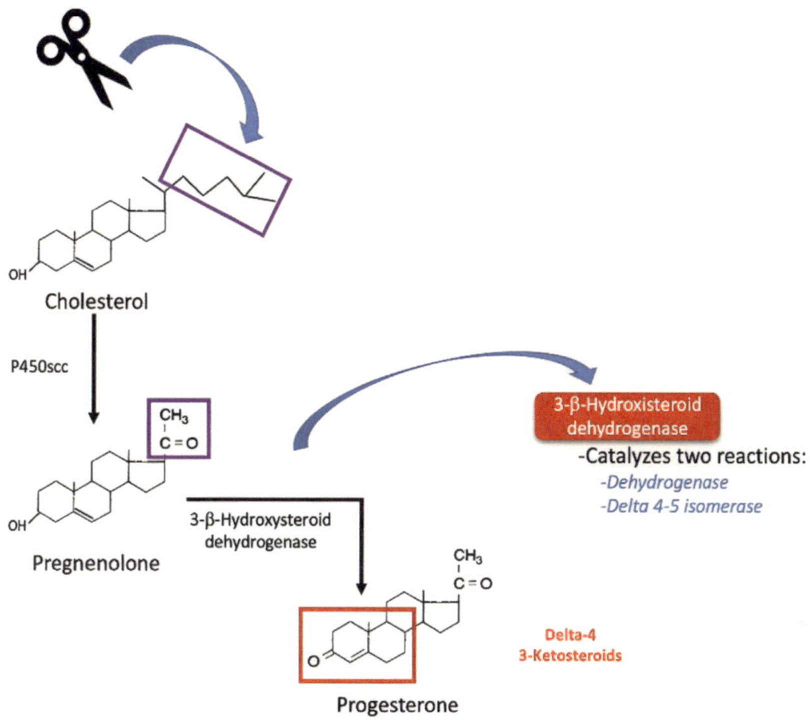

Figure 1.
Progesterone synthesis [1].

Progestins have a longer duration of action and are more stable than natural progesterone, so they are utilised in therapeutics [1]. They act by binding to nuclear receptors; therefore, the processes they may influence are very broad and include the regulation of endometrium, the activity of glands, and even reproduction [7]. Progestins serve various purposes, including their use in contraception methods such as progestin-only pills and in the treatment of gynaecological disorders like endometriosis [2].

2.1.2 Development of progestins

García-Sáenz et al. [1] give the historical development of progestins; this covers the period from the discovery of the ovarian corpus luteum and its association with pregnancy. CL was first described by Gabriele Falloppio in the mid-1500s, while in 1672, Regnier de Graaf described the ovarian follicle. In 1896, Emil Knauer extended his work on the association between the CL and pregnancy. By 1929, George W. Corner and Willard M. Allen successfully isolated a compound from porcine CL, identified by the chemical formula C21H30O2, which they named "progestin" due to its pregnancy-supporting properties (See **Figure 2**) [1].

In 1934, Corner and Allen produced crystalline progestin in the U.S., while European researchers, including Adolf Butenandt, independently synthesised the same compound. Butenandt's work, which detailed the delta-4-3-ketosteroid structure, earned him the Nobel Prize in Chemistry in 1939. Although there was debate over naming the hormone "luteosterone" due to its origin in the CL, the term "progesterone" (P4) became the accepted name [1].

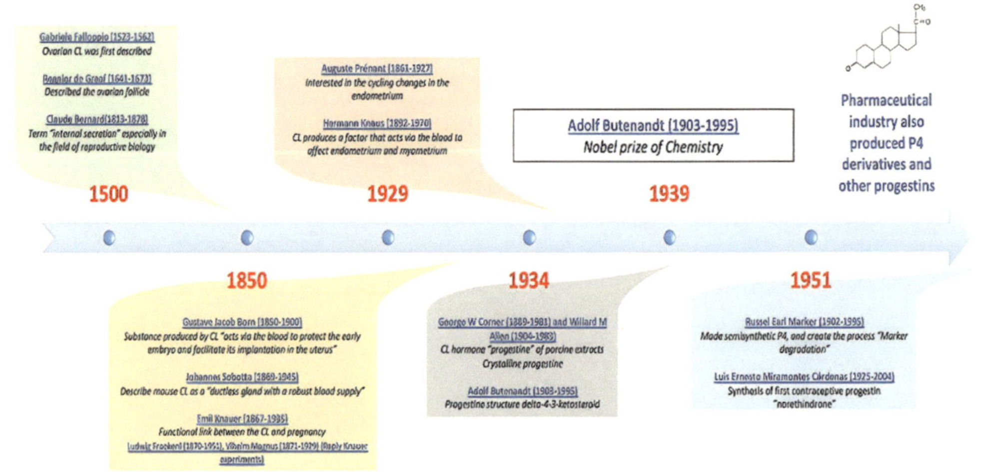

Figure 2.
Timeline for progestin development [1].

Russell Marker made a significant breakthrough in 1943 by developing the "Marker degradation" method, which enabled P4 extraction from plant materials, facilitating the large-scale production of synthetic hormones. In 1951, Marker, while working in Mexico, synthesised P4 from diosgenin derived from Dioscorea plant roots and founded the Syntex laboratory. During the same year, Luis Miramontes created norethindrone, the first orally active synthetic progestin, though it was not initially tested for contraceptive use [1].

Progestins' contraceptive effects were later confirmed when Gregory Pincus demonstrated that high doses of P4 could inhibit ovulation by suppressing gonadotropin release. In 1951, Pincus tested P4 in women, though the results were initially inconsistent. Further research led to the development of norethynodrel, a 19-nor steroid shown to be an effective contraceptive by Pincus, John Rock, and Celso-Ramón García when used correctly by women [1].

Due to their wide application in contraception throughout the 1950s and 1960s, progestins expanded their use outside of birth control. New synthetic progestins with improved properties were found through continued research and are currently used to treat several reproductive endocrine diseases, such as endometriosis and polycystic ovary syndrome, making progestins an essential factor in fertility [1].

2.1.3 Mechanisms of progestins actions

According to Song and Fraser [5], and further elaborated by Malik and Nadeem [8], the mechanism of action of progestins was explained in terms of interaction with specific nuclear receptors, notably the progesterone receptors. These exist mainly in two forms: progesterone receptor A (PR-A) and progesterone receptor B (PR-B). These receptors differ in their functions and are expressed differently within tissues. Such receptors transmit the action of the progestins as a DNA-interacting complex, which may stimulate or repress gene activity. The responses of the endometrium to such an interacting complex include the inhibition of glandular growth, decidualisation of stroma, and infiltration by leukocytes [5, 8].

Exogenous progestins represent the artificial variants of natural progesterone [5]. Their action is divergent from the action of endogenous progesterone secreted by the ovaries. They act via a modulating effect at the hypothalamic-pituitary-ovarian axis by reducing the secretion of gonadotropin-releasing hormone and, therefore, preventing action on ovulation. Their main action in the endometrium will be to prepare or inhibit its receptivity for the implantation of the embryo, according to the purpose of contraception [8].

Progestins are categorised based on their progestational, anti-estrogenic, and anti-androgenic effects [9]. These effects are critical to their contraceptive uses as well as their disease state indications, such as endometriosis. Progestational effects enable the transformation of the endometrium into the secretory stage of the menstrual cycle, preparing the uterus for pregnancy. Anti-estrogenic effects thin the oestrogen-primed endometrium. Anti-androgenic effects inhibit testosterone by blocking access to androgen receptors (AR) [10].

In addition to these genomic effects of progestins, rapid, non-genomic effects occur via mechanisms that do not involve classical nuclear receptors. These are mediated by a number of membrane-bound receptors, including progestin and adipoQ receptors (PAQRs) and the progesterone receptor membrane component 1 (PGRMC1) [1]. These other modes of action lead to modifications in cellular Ca^{2+} flux, production of cyclic adenosine monophosphate (cAMP), and neuroprotection. These pathways are involved in numerous processes: the maturation of the oocyte, immune modulation, and protection against cell death. The use of androgen receptors (AR), glucocorticoid receptors (GR), and mineralocorticoid receptors (MR), however, leads to side effects that include acne, increases in lipids, and fluid retention [11].

2.1.4 Classification of progestins

2.1.4.1 Chemical/structural classification of progestins

Progestins are generically divided based on their molecular structure, which defines their potency and pharmacokinetic profile. Progestogenic activity depends on the presence of a 3-keto group and a double bond between carbon (C) 4 and C5 in the A ring (Δ4-3-keto group) [12]. Progestins without this structure (desogestrel or norgestimate) are prodrugs and must be converted into active metabolites following oral administration [1].

Progestins can loosely be grouped into four categories based on their structural relationship to either progesterone (P4) or testosterone (T), including pregnanes, norpregnanes, estranes, and gonanes (See **Figures 3–8** below) [1, 13].

1. *Pregnanes:* This includes all progestins related to P4 with a methyl group at the C10 position [1, 14].

2. *Norpregnanes:* These progestins are derived from 19-norprogesterone and are characterised by the absence of a methyl group at C10 or the lack of a C19 group. Some norpregnanes may contain an acetate group, while others do not [1, 14].

3. *Estranes:* Estranes are related to testosterone and are identified as ethinylated progestins due to the absence of an ethyl group at the C13 position [1, 9].

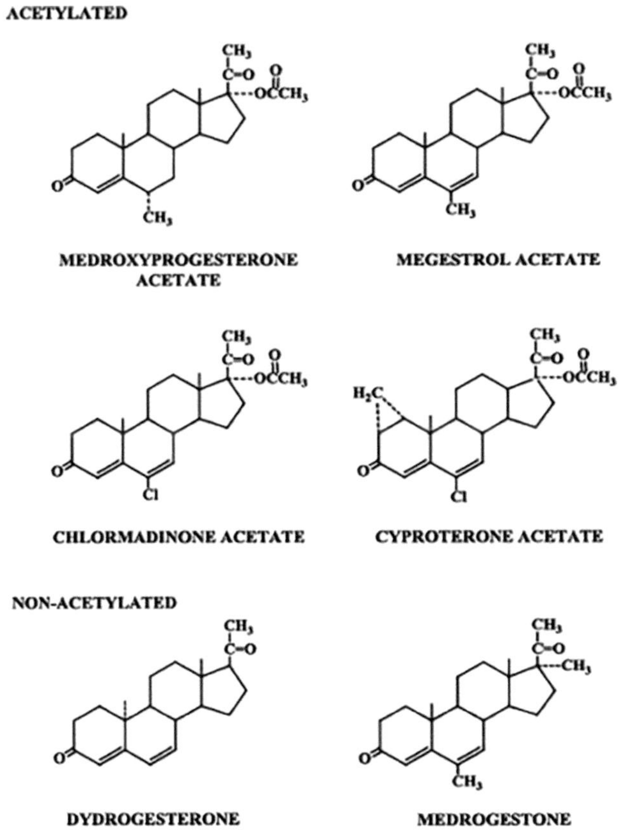

Figure 3.
Derivatives of pregnane [13].

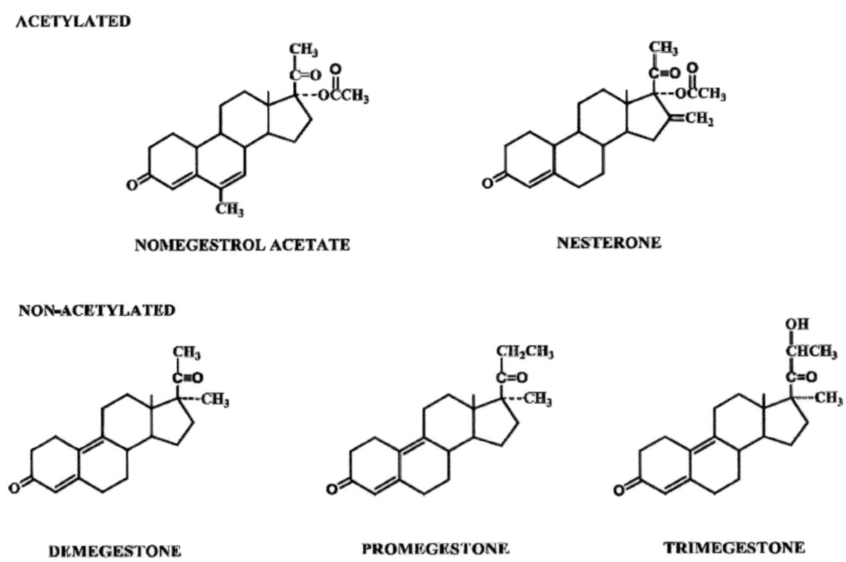

Figure 4.
Derivatives of Norpregnanes [13].

DOI: http://dx.doi.org/10.5772/intechopen.1007931

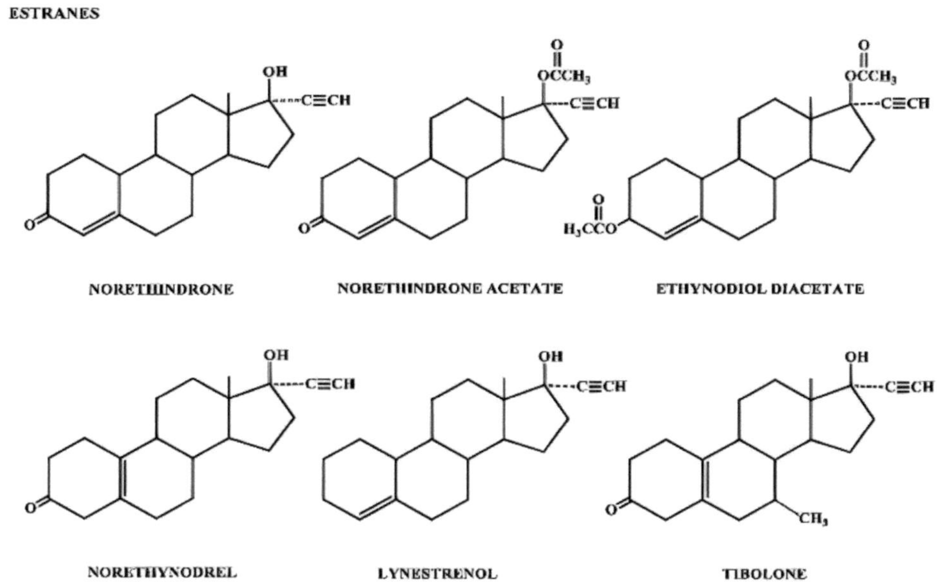

Figure 5.
Estranes as ethinylated derivatives [13].

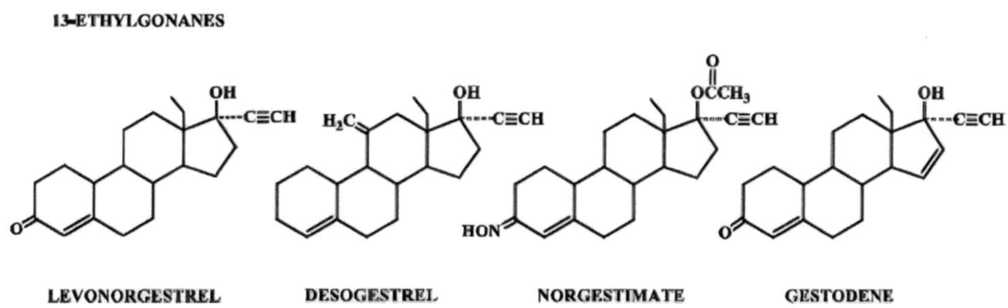

Figure 6.
13-ethylgonanes as ethinylated derivatives [13].

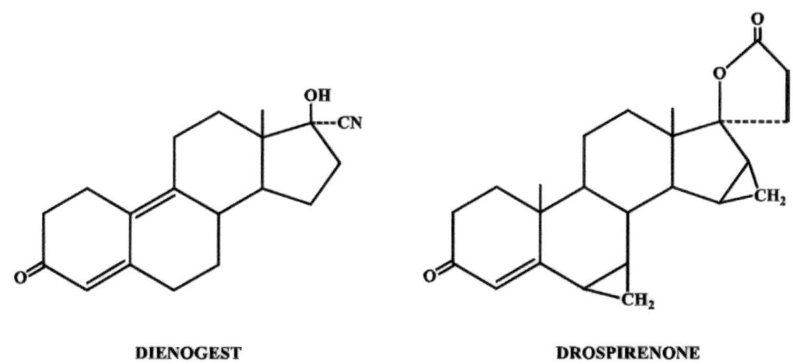

Figure 7.
Non-ethyl derivatives [13].

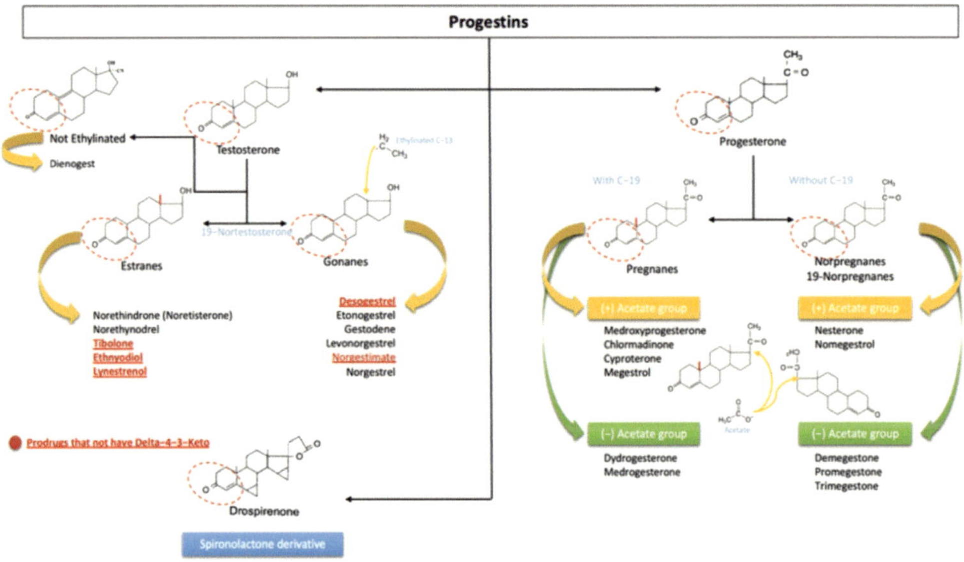

Figure 8.
Overall classification of Progestins based on their chemical structures [1].

4. *Gonanes:* This group includes 13-ethylgonanes, which have an ethyl group at the C13 position of the steroid structure [1, 9].

5. *Non-ethyl groups:* Some progestins may not have an ethyl group, which further differentiates them. These structural variations are essential for understanding various progestins' unique effects and applications in clinical settings.

The dotted lines indicate the necessary Δ4-3-Keto group required for binding to the progesterone receptor while also highlighting the general structural differences at C19 and C13 across various types of progestins. Red underlined labels represent prodrugs lacking the classical Δ4–3-Keto group, including the distinctive spironolactone derivative. It is important to note that each molecule within the same group has unique properties, although their individual structures are not displayed [1].

2.1.4.2 Generative structure (other classification of progestin)

In addition to chemical classification, progestins are categorised based on their generation and derivative structure [9]. This classification provides insights into their pharmacological properties and potential side effects [1]. The classification is as follows:

2.1.4.2.1 Based on generations

1. *Older progestins:* It includes the First (1st), Second (2nd), and Third (3rd) generations, most of which are derived from testosterone, leading to androgenic effects. They are predominantly derivatives of 19-nortestosterone. Some are derived from pregnanes or 17-hydroxyprogesterone [1, 9, 15].

2. *Newer progestins:* The Fourth (4th) generation is designed to closely resemble natural progesterone, reducing androgenic, estrogenic, mineralocorticoid, and

glucocorticoid side effects. The fourth progestins are derivatives of the 19-norprogesterone or nor-pregnane, which are created to minimise unwanted side effects.

3. *Exceptions:* There are exceptions in these generations, such as the Dienogest (A derivative of ethylated 19-nortestosterone) and Drospirenone (A spironolactone derivative)

This generational classification is useful for understanding the evolution of progestin development and its varied biological impacts (**Figure 9**).

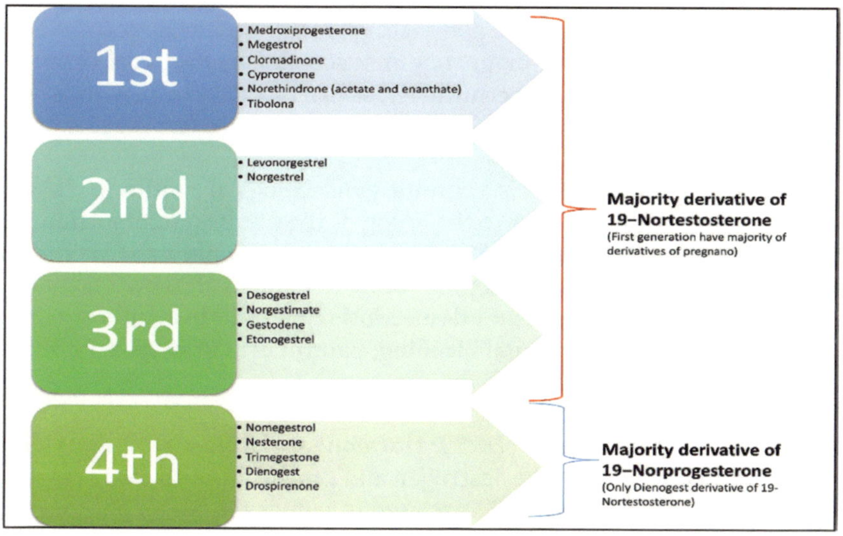

Figure 9.
Generational classification of progestins [1].

2.2 Role of progestins in female reproductive health and therapeutics

Progestins play significant roles in reproduction and in various clinical applications because of their endometrial effects [1, 5]. These include menstruation, ovulation, pregnancy, contraception, and gynaecological conditions like endometriosis, as well as hormone replacement therapy and assisted reproductive techniques [1]. Each of the reproductive health conditions, procedures, and outcomes is described below:

1. *Menstruation:* Menstruation is the natural monthly process in which the uterine lining is shed, leading to bleeding that usually lasts from 3 to 7 days. The menstrual cycle, typically around 28 days in length, can vary from person to person [1]. In other words, menstruation marks a failure to achieve conception and the need to shed the specialised uterine lining, which is caused mainly by the withdrawal of progesterone [16].

2. *Ovulation*: Ovulation can be defined as the biological process in the female reproductive cycle when an ovum (mature egg) is released from one of the ovaries into the fallopian tube, where it might eventually be fertilised by sperm. It usually occurs in the middle of the menstrual cycle (i.e. 14th day of a 28-day cycle). This stage is vital for fertility as it signifies the best time for conception [17].

3. *Pregnancy:* Pregnancy commences when a fertilised egg implants into the uterine wall, leading to the development of an embryo and eventually a foetus over a period of around 40 weeks [18]. *Pregnancy* can be defined as the state of having the products of conception (such as an embryo or foetus) implanted within the uterus or elsewhere in the body (as in ectopic pregnancy, where implantation takes place outside the uterus) [19].

4. *Contraception:* The term contraception refers to a range of techniques used to avoid pregnancy. Hormonal contraceptives, like progestins, are highly successful in preventing pregnancy. They operate by controlling ovulation and changing cervical mucus to prevent sperm from penetrating [4, 20]. Contraception also refers to the intentional prevention of pregnancy or conception by the use of various devices (e.g., IUDs), chemicals (e.g., spermicides), sexual practices (e.g., withdrawal method), drugs (e.g., birth control pills), or surgical procedures (e.g., vasectomy) [21].

5. *Endometriosis:* Endometriosis is a chronic gynaecological condition characterised by the growth of tissue similar to the lining of the uterus (endometrium) outside the uterine cavity. The misplaced endometrial tissue (glands and/or stroma) can be found on the ovaries, fallopian tubes, the outer surface of the uterus, or other organs within the pelvis. Endometriosis can result in symptoms like pelvic discomfort, excessive menstrual bleeding, painful urination/defecation and difficulties with fertility [1, 22, 23].

6. *Hormone replacement therapy (HRT):* Hormone replacement therapy (HRT) includes giving hormones like oestrogen and progesterone to ease symptoms of menopause. Progestins in HRT are used to reduce the risk of endometrial hyperplasia and address the potential dangers of using oestrogen therapy alone [20]. Hormone replacement therapy (HRT) is also referred to as a treatment used to replenish women with ovarian hormones lost during the transition to menopause, specifically oestrogen and progesterone, to alleviate symptoms associated with menopause [24].

7. *Assisted reproductive techniques (ART):* Assisted reproductive technology (ART) refers to medical procedures used to treat infertility by handling either eggs or embryos outside the female's body [25]. Assisted reproductive technology encompasses procedures like in vitro fertilisation (IVF) and fertility drugs that aim to improve the chances of conception by encouraging ovulation and assisting in the fertilisation process [18].

The specific roles of progestin are discussed for each of the female reproductive health and therapeutic conditions as follows.

2.2.1 Role of progestins in menstruation

Progestins are artificial derivatives of the naturally occurring steroid hormone, progesterone, which have critical roles in maintaining menstrual cyclicity and in conditions associated with reproduction. They greatly affect endometrial function, menstrual bleeding, and overall hormonal balance [1, 2]. Existing studies have identified the specific roles of progestins in menstruation. This section synthesises those studies to highlight the roles of progestins in menstruation (**Figure 10**).

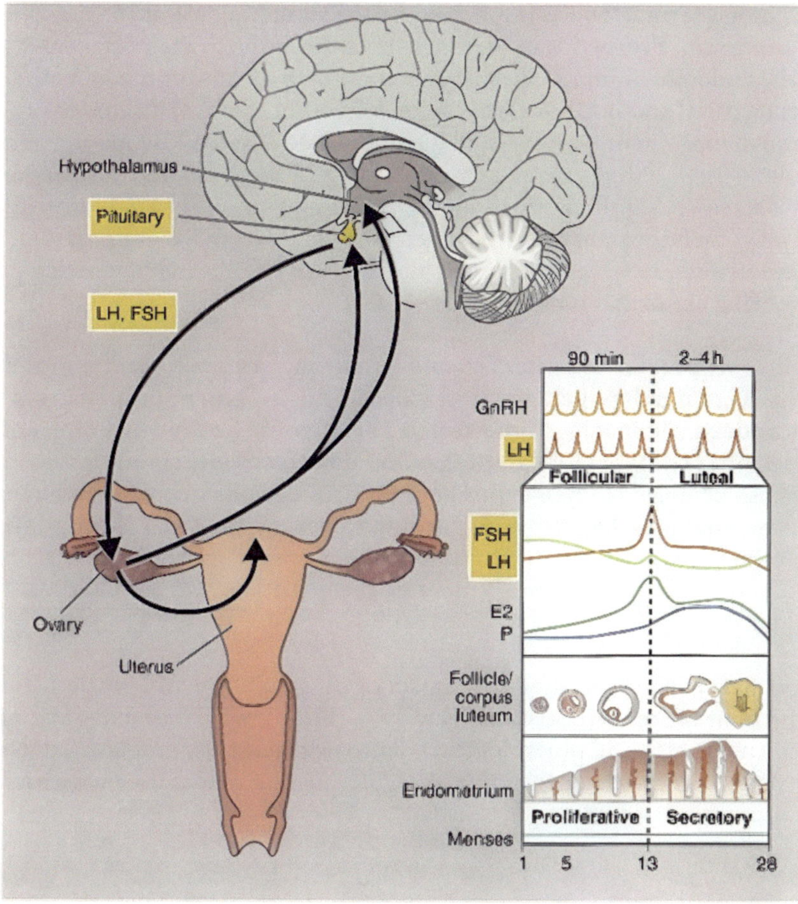

Figure 10.
Anatomy and physiology of the menstrual cycle [26].

1. *Endometrial preparation and maintenance:* Progestins are a major constituent in the menstrual cycle, mimicking the effect of natural progesterone, especially during the luteal phase [26]. Following ovulation, the corpus luteum secretes progesterone to prepare the endometrium lining for embryo implantation [26]. During the luteal phase, progestins play a role similar to natural progesterone by preparing the endometrial lining for potential implantation. This effect is vital in hormonal therapies designed to support fertility or manage menstrual irregularities. Schatz et al. [27] describe the mechanism of how progestins upregulate the expression of tissue factors in endometrial stromal cells. The tissue factor is an important step in homeostasis and the maintenance of the endometrium. Its expression is induced by progestin, thereby playing a role in maintaining the endometrium in a steady state and allowing embryo implantation. The latter again points out the role of progestins in providing a favourable environment for early pregnancy. Thus reducing the likelihood of early pregnancy loss [27].

2. *Regulation of menstrual bleeding:* Progestins also play significant roles in the regulation of menstrual bleeding. Menstrual bleeding is a result of withdrawal

from progesterone, which is followed by the sloughing off of the lining of the endometrium. Progestins reduce menstrual flow due to their effect of stabilising the endometrium; these characteristics form a basis for many methods of contraception and hormonal therapies. Vercellini et al. [3] discussed progestins for the management of menstrual disorders associated with menorrhagia and dysmenorrhea. Progestins stabilise the lining of the endometrium, and hence, flow decreases, significantly reducing the symptoms of menstruation [3]. This role plays an important part in women who suffer from a condition such as endometriosis, in which progestins alleviate the condition by reducing pain and preventing abnormal tissue growth.

3. *Regulation of menstrual disorders and managing menstrual health:* Progestins have gained much popularity nowadays in the treatment of menstrual disorders. Indeed, their role is time-tested in controlling heavy bleeding and painful periods [1]. In particular, progestins act effectively against endometriosis, a disease wherein women experience painful periods due to abnormal growth of tissues outside the uterus. According to Vercellini et al. [3], progestins induce atrophy of the endometrium and suppress abnormal growth of tissues, hence relief and improvement of the quality of life among the affected women.

   Elliott-Sale et al. [7] studied the impact of progestins on athletic performance throughout the menstrual cycle. However, their significance in maintaining menstrual health and physiological balance was not fully emphasised. Nevertheless, progestins play a crucial role in regulating and managing menstrual health conditions.

4. *Induction of menstruation:* Progestins also act to induce menstruation in cases of amenorrhea. This will be helpful for those women who experience amenorrhea due to hormonal imbalances or disorders that affect the normal menstrual cycle. Progestins mimic the cycle's luteal phase by stimulating the shedding of the endometrium to induce menstruation. Berga and Johnston-MacAnanny [26] review physiological processes that are modulated by progestins and indicate their use both in the maintenance of regular cycles and the treatment of disorders resulting from hormonal imbalance. Thus, their study justifies the clinical application of progestins for inducing menses and treating menstrual disorders [26].

5. *Progestin's role in hormonal balance during menstruation:* Progestin stabilises the almost-continuous hormonal fluctuations throughout the menstrual cycle. Such fluctuations in hormones can cause irregular cycles, mood swings, and, most especially, changes during the premenstrual part of the cycle. Progestins counteract excessive oestrogen effects, thus providing a more regulated hormonal environment. Avila-Varela et al. [28] reviewed how hormonal changes throughout the menstrual cycle led to variations in brain activity and network dynamics. The study highlighted the role that progestins, among other hormones, play in modulating neural processes and general brain functioning [28]. In these ways, progestins stabilise these hormonal changes so as not to disrupt cognitive and emotional functioning.

6. *Progestin role in brain dynamics:* Recent studies have shown that progestins alter brain activities and network dynamics throughout the menstrual cycle. Elliott-Sale et al. [7] showed that progestins are relevant in maintaining the physiologic conditions of athlete women's menstrual cycles and overall well-being. Avila-Varela et al. [28] found that varied levels of progestins have implications for the complexity of reconfiguration and brain network. These findings provide further consequences for the role of progestins in physiological and psychological well-being.

7. *Concern for progestins roles in menstruation:* Progestins have been identified to be medically significant in regulating menstrual bleeding, menstrual disorders treatments, and inducing menstruation. However, safety and long-term effects continue to be researched. According to Vercellini et al. [3], despite the efficiency of progestins, they cannot be suggested for every woman, especially in cases of progesterone resistance. Besides, the risk of abnormal uterine bleeding following long-term therapy with progestins, noted by Schatz et al. [27], needs very attentive monitoring and treatment individualised for each woman. Also, Grindlay et al. [29] were concerned about the current over-the-counter approval of progestin-only pills and discussed more questions about accessibility and further research into the broader implications of such a product, are created. In addition, Bonnema and Dalebout [30] stated that the abuse of high-dose oestrogen/progestin combinations indicates cultural and regional differences in the use of hormone drugs, which they attributed to cultural and regional factors. The use is abusive or inappropriate in certain regions and might bring harmful side effects to the user [30]. This again brings to light that education and proper legislation will go a long way in ensuring safety and efficacy in using progestins. Despite all these concerns raised by existing studies regarding the progestins' roles in menstruation, it has proven to be useful in regulating menstrual bleeding, menstrual disorders treatments, and inducing menstruation

In summary, progestins play a multidimensional role in menstruation and reproductive health. These after-effects are well established regarding endometrial preparation, menstrual bleeding, and hormonal balance and are supported by recent studies. Given that the benefits of progestins are so remarkably considerable in menstrual disorder management and hormonal fluctuation, continuous research is still necessary to tackle safety issues and improve their use for diverse populations. As progestin knowledge is continuously updated, so will their application in reproductive health advance and improve outcomes for women of reproductive age worldwide.

2.2.2 Role of progestins in ovulation

Progestins are an essential factor in regulating ovulation, whether spontaneous or through medical intervention, due to their significant effect on the surge release of the luteinizing hormone responsible for inducing ovulation. Thus, their use has varied from contraception and hormone therapies to, more recently, assisted reproductive technologies by providing these inhibiting, delaying, or suppressing actions on ovulation. However, their role in ovulation is not confined to ART; they are involved in significant ways at several levels in the natural cycle and in general reproductive health.

1. *Progestin as an Ovulation Inhibitor:* Perhaps the most fundamental action of progestin in inhibiting ovulation is its ability to block the surge of Luteinizing hormone (LH). Luteinising hormone (LH), released from the anterior pituitary, is crucial for triggering ovulation by causing mature follicles in the ovary to rupture. Progestin inhibits this process by acting on the hypothalamic-pituitary-gonadal axis, suppressing the release of GnRH from the hypothalamus. This results in reduced secretion of pituitary luteinizing hormone (LH) and follicle-stimulating hormone (FSH), preventing ovulation. This is one of the suppressive actions that progestin performs on LH as a way of preventing ovulation and pregnancy when using a progestin-only contraceptive.

   Pelican et al. [31] reported that progestin is highly effective in suppressing ovarian activity, thereby synchronising the oestrous cycle of cats. Treatment resulted in an improved ovarian response to exogenous gonadotropins due to the predictable timing of ovulation. This high level of effectiveness is vital in managing spontaneous and induced ovulators and provides a reliable technique for controlling reproductive cycles for various species.

   Storer et al. [32] demonstrated that progestins significantly regulate the reproductive cycle. Their study found that sustained-release progestin products, of which altrenogest is one, suppressed estrus and delayed ovulation in mares. This study finding is relevant to regulating the reproductive cycle over extended periods and is an essential veterinary use of progestins irrespective of a human model.

   The investigation by Endrikat et al. [33] focused on how progestin works in preventing follicular growth and ovulation within different contraceptive products. Progestins remain among the cornerstones of contraceptive methods, and the results of all such studies confirm that a steady level of the hormone inhibits ovulation. The present study again confirms the established role of progestin in contraception in assuring reliable ovulation inhibition across different dosages and formulations.

   Further, La Marca and Capuzzo [34] conclude that progestins are among the most favourite drugs for preventing spontaneous ovulation during ovarian stimulation since they do not affect oocyte quality negatively due to surge prevention of LH and premature ovulation. Other contraceptive forms include progestin-only pills, intrauterine devices, and injectable forms, which act primarily by preventing ovulation through the hormone. These contraceptives prevent the development of a dominant follicle and the LH surge necessary for ovulation by maintaining a steady level of progestin and creating a hormonal environment that is not conducive to such developments. In essence, the constant presence of progestin tricks the body into believing that the luteal phase of a menstrual cycle is occurring, and hence, no further follicular development will occur.

   Cosentino et al. [35] noted that pre-treatment with progestins in Saanen goats successfully synchronised ovulation and, importantly, reduced variability in the timing of ovulation. This was advantageous to the fixed-time artificial insemination (FTAI) and superovulation (SOV) protocols. Progestin administration allowed better control over ovarian activity to ensure predictable ovulation, a necessary condition for timed insemination in both human and veterinary reproductive treatments.

Xie et al. [36] extended the molecular basis of this action by showing that progestin downregulates luteinizing hormone (LH) expression and its receptors, luteinizing hormone/chorionic gonadotropin receptor (LHCGR), on preovulatory follicles, thereby lowering progesterone synthesis and extending the timing of ovulation. In reproductive medicine, progestins are utilised to prevent spontaneous ovulation by blocking the LH surge during ovarian stimulation.

2. *Delay of ovulation in progestin-primed ovarian stimulation (PPOS):* Progestin partially disrupts the usual physiologic sequence, leading to follicular rupture and thus delaying ovulation. Xie et al. [36] demonstrate that PPOS suppresses ovulation through downregulation of crucial genes critical in this process, which are luteinizing hormone/chorionic gonadotropin receptor (LHCGR), A disintegrin and metalloproteinase with thrombospondin motifs 1 (ADAMTS-1), and vascular endothelial growth factor A (VEGF-A). These genes play a critical role in the process of follicular rupture. Progestin interferes with these pathways, blocking LH secretion and causing the egg to be released considerably later than otherwise. The fine-tuning of the timing of ovulation also extends the possibilities of applications in fertility preservation and contraception procedures, as many rely on the proper timing of ovulation for their effectiveness.

3. *Progestin in the luteal phase and endometrial receptivity after ovulation:* The corpus luteum produces progesterone, which thickens the endometrium lining in preparation for embryo implantation. Progestin is, therefore, a synthetic derivative or analogue of progesterone, playing this role in hormone therapies and certain reproductive procedures. As in natural cycles, progestin lengthens the luteal phase in these cases in a way that maintains the receptiveness of the endometrium to the fertilised egg. Its importance during this stage has been further echoed in works such as Takahashi and Ogiwara [37], in which it was said that progestin receptors were important for the rupture of follicles in vertebrates. These authors reported LH surge induces progestin receptor expression in granulosa cells.

4. *Progestin and LH surge modulation in clinical practice:* The modulation of the LH surge is a core function of progestin in natural as well as medically managed cycles. Examples of these technologies include fertility preservation technologies and hormonal treatments for polycystic ovary syndrome (PCOS) and endometriosis that use progestin to induce or suppress ovulation on time. Chen et al. [38] conducted a randomised trial. The results showed comparable live birth rates and embryo quality between progestin-primed ovarian stimulation and GnRH antagonist protocols, thus proving that progestin can effectively modulate ovulation in ART and natural cycles.

5. *Progestin use facilitates medical protocols economically and logistically:* Progestin used for ovulatory suppression has practical advantages in the medical arena, reducing clinical visits and injections needed in treatments like IVF. Goodman et al. [39] proved that progestin suppression during oocyte cryopreservation decreases patients' logistical and financial burdens without significantly diminishing the number or quality of oocytes retrieved. This also indicates various

useful applications of progestin in regulating ovulation and managing patients by simplifying the treatment modalities. The versatility of progestin, as various studies cited concerning ovulation, speaks to natural and assisted reproductive procedures.

6. *Regulation of Oocyte maturation and ovulation:* Wu et al. [40] point out that the major actor of oocyte maturation is progestin through membrane progestin receptors (mPRs). In zebrafish, the knockout model for mPRs showed defects in oocyte maturation. Their ovulation was retarded significantly; therefore, their fertility was very poor. Progestin influences nuclear progestin receptors (Pgr), which are involved in ovulation. This finding underlines that progestin signalling pathways are important in regulating the timing of ovulation and the full maturation of oocytes, which is important for successful fertilisation.

7. *Improved ovulation induction outcomes:* The study conducted by Cai et al. [41] focused on the induction of ovulation of poor ovarian responders by progestins, especially medroxyprogesterone acetate, either in in vitro fertilisation (IVF) or intracytoplasmic sperm injection (ICSI) treatments. In addition, the protocol of Progestin-Primed Ovarian Stimulation (PPOS) reduces the cancellation rate and increases the recovery of mature oocytes, enhancing the quality of the embryos. In the PPOS protocol, external progesterone is administered to suppress the release of LH in the early follicular phase, helping to maintain a consistent hormonal environment for the maturation of oocytes [42]. This could be another role of progestin in managing hard-to-treat patients and improving fertility outcomes from ART.

Therefore, progestin predominantly hinders the LH surge, which is crucial for follicular rupture. Its uses span from natural reproductive health to contraception and medical interventions, making it a versatile tool for regulating ovulation timing, improving endometrial receptivity, and achieving more favourable clinical results. Progestin plays a vital role in reproductive medicine due to its demonstrated capacity, as shown in several studies, to hinder, delay, or precisely regulate ovulation.

2.2.3 Role of progestins in pregnancy

The following discussion explores the role of progestins in pregnancy based on findings from existing studies. These are geared at delineating the role of progestin in unintended pregnancies, ectopic pregnancy, abnormal pregnancy diagnosis, prevention against preterm birth, and risks associated with hypospadias.

1. *Prevention against unintended pregnancies:* Progestin plays a vital role in preventing pregnancy, particularly when used in progestin-only pills, injectables, and implants. A study by Guillard et al. [43] shows that over-the-counter progestin-only pills (OTC POPs) can make quite an impact in reducing unintended pregnancies. Their model estimates that assuming exclusive use of OTC POPs, the net reduction would amount to 30,624 unintended pregnancies annually. This supports the potential benefit of increasing access to progestin-based contraception, as increased access may actually help women avoid unplanned pregnancies-a great public health concern. Wollum et al. [44] similarly emphasised the cost of the use of progestin-based contraception by modelling the effect that reduction

or complete elimination of the out-of-pocket price of POPs would have in terms of wider diffusion of the method, especially within low-income populations. Thus, progestin's effectiveness will sooner or later be influenced by how accessible and affordable it is. In both studies, progestin has been highlighted as a crucial factor in leaving the decision of reproduction to women, especially in resource-poor countries where not everyone can afford more expensive means of contraception.

2. *Risk of ectopic pregnancy:* Progestin-only injectables and implants are rare to fail as methods of contraception. However, in those very rare chances of failure, Callahan et al. [45] were able to show a risk for ectopic pregnancies. The systematic review reflects that the progestin methods carry a slightly higher risk of ectopic pregnancies compared to the other contraceptives; however, this risk is minimal, considering their overall effectiveness. Therefore, this calls for patient education and counselling about the associated risks with progestin-only contraceptives, thus ensuring that users make an informed decision.

3. *Maintenance of uterine quiescence and prevention of preterm birth (maintenance of pregnancy):* Progestin maintains pregnancy, suppresses inflammatory signals, and inhibits uterine contractions [46]. Progesterone, a natural progestin, maintains an intrauterine environment and prevents preterm labour, which is one of the leading causes of neonatal morbidity and mortality. It was also evidenced in the study that synthetic progestins, such dydrogesterone are clinically used to prevent preterm birth in cases of women with a previous history of preterm deliveries [47, 48]. Byrns [46] also highlights that different progestins act through different mechanisms, determining the effectiveness of progestin in maintaining uterine quiescence. Supporting that, each progestin therapy needs to be tailored based on individual cases, considering the type of progestin used and the specific risk factors involved in each pregnancy.

4. *Reconstituting hormonal status in jeopardised pregnancies (maintenance of pregnancy):* Shikichi et al. [49] provided an added critical dimension to the role of progestin in pregnancy by focusing on its diagnostic and therapeutic use in managing abnormal pregnancies. The study conducted on mares shows that deviations in progestin levels can serve as a signal for compromised pregnancies, and treatment with progestin helps restore hormonal balance for better outcomes in pregnancy. Mares treated for low levels of progestin had significantly higher survival rates for their foals, thus suggesting that progestin supplementation could be a critical determinant in pregnancy loss prevention. Even though this study is within the veterinary context, the results applicable to human pregnancies are that close hormonal monitoring with timely progestin intervention in high-risk pregnancies improves maternity and foetal outcomes.

5. *Progestin causes hypospadias as a developmental risk in pregnancy:* though progestin is an essential drug in the course of pregnancies, there are some possible risks associated with it. Akay and Yıldız [50] conducted research and found that maternal exposure to progestins has been related to the development of hypospadias, a congenital anomaly of the urethra, in male offspring. In a retrospective case-control study, they identified that prolonged progestin exposure during pregnancy, especially among women with high-risk occupational groups

exposed to endocrine disruptors, was significantly associated with an increased risk of hypospadias. The above findings raised important questions, especially regarding the teratogenic action of synthetic progestins in the event of excessive use or under particular exposure conditions. For those situations where progestin is indispensable in specific contexts of pregnancy management, this research suggests that caution needs to be exercised with respect to such use in a more protracted or high-dose manner, especially in populations that may be exposed to other risk factors.

6. *Progestin as a hormonal diagnostic tool in managing pregnancy outcomes:* Beyond the application of progestin in therapeutics, it could serve as a very useful diagnostic biomarker related to pregnancy health. The application of progestin and oestrogen levels was done by Shikichi et al. [49] to monitor foetal-placenta function at late gestation. The study reported that lower levels of progestin are associated with higher incidences of foal loss, whereas their normalisation following treatment is associated with healthy delivery. It would, therefore, indicate that progestin measurements could be used in human obstetric care, where, through monitoring of hormonal profiles, early detection of at-risk pregnancies could be made and intervention provided in good time. In this direction, progestin could be used more comprehensively in diagnostic protocols concerning high-risk pregnancies. It could be considered for improving outcomes through early detection and management of the condition.

The reviewed studies point toward the multifaceted nature of progestin's role in pregnancy, depicting its therapeutic value and associated risks. While Guillard et al. [43] and Wollum et al. [44] discuss the benefits of hormonal contraception, especially in access and affordability, the discussion by Byrns [46] and Shikichi et al. [49] primarily highlights the role this birth control plays in preventing preterm birth and the handling of abnormal pregnancies. On the other hand, it was also shown in works by Callahan et al. [45] and Akay and Yıldız [50] that progestin, though effective, is not free of complications, including increased slight risks for ectopic pregnancies and developmental anomalies such as hypospadias. Therefore, progestins have a dual role in pregnancy outcomes, with benefits and risks that have to be weighed. The wide application of unwanted pregnancy prevention to the maintenance of hormonal stability necessary for sustaining a pregnancy makes this modality an indispensable tool in reproductive health. Caution is needed in patient selection and follow-up to reduce its risks.

2.2.4 Role of progestins in contraception

This section discusses progestins' roles in contraception under different themes highlighted using evidence from existing studies.

1. *Bleeding control in progestin-based contraceptives:* The role of progestin in regulating and controlling bleeding is critical to its efficacy and acceptability as a choice for contraception. Shoupe [51] indicates that progestin-based methods, such as hormonal IUDs and progestin-dominant oral contraceptives that suppress ovulation, have been able to manage heavy menstrual bleeding with its accompanying irregular bleeding patterns. These effectively prevent acute heavy bleeding and maintain long-term bleeding control. The Shoupe study [51] underlines the

benefits of MPA, which does not convert to ethinyl estradiol, thus minimising the risk of side effects. However, in a randomised clinical trial, Edelman et al. [52] evaluated the effect of curcumin on bleeding patterns associated with the use of the etonogestrel implant. They concluded that this agent had no significant impact on improving bleeding control. Thus, while progestin-only contraceptives may often result in bleeding control, ancillary treatments like curcumin may not improve bleeding control in all users. This finding points to the multifactorial nature of progestin-related bleeding, where disrupted angiogenesis and inflammation are among the mechanisms involved.

2. *Endometrial modulation by progestin:* Progestin's ability to modulate the endometrium is a linchpin to its contraceptive effect. In those patients seeking an alternative to surgical options, this is the most valuable aspect of progestin. Mandelbaum et al. [53] discuss obese women with complex atypical hyperplasia, comparing levonorgestrel (LNG) and intrauterine device (IUD) versus systemic progestin therapy. Their findings indicate that local progestin therapy with the LNG-IUD affords superior endometrial modulation, as manifested by a higher rate of complete response and decreased risk of progression to cancer, especially among morbidly obese women. The above study illustrates that local progestin delivery may provide more specific and adequate endometrial protection, especially in women with particular health challenges like obesity. Systemic progestin is less optimum than the focused action of the LNG-IUD.

3. *Impact of progestin on ovarian reserve:* Hariton et al. [54] studied the link between contraceptive use and Anti-Müllerian Hormone (AMH) levels, an indirect indicator of ovarian reserve. The study found that using hormonal contraceptives, especially those containing progestin, is linked to lower average AMH levels compared to women not using contraception. This association was consistent across different progestin methods, such as implants, hormonal IUDs, and progestin-only pills. The practical implication of this finding is that while progestin contraceptives are effective, they can make it more complicated to interpret ovarian reserve test results. However, this effect does not seem to have a long-term impact on fertility, as AMH levels typically recover after stopping hormonal contraception.

4. *Contraceptive efficacy and satisfaction:* Among the most effective ways of contraception, implants, IUDs, and oral pills containing progestin only have been proven. Edelman et al. (49) provide data on the etonogestrel implant. Despite issues with the bleeding pattern, this implant has proven to be effective and well-accepted for contraception. Generally, progestin-contraceptive methods are associated with high satisfaction, as documented by clinical and observational studies, though individual experiences with side effects such as irregular bleeding may impact continuation rates. In addition, Shoupe [51] reiterates the effectiveness of progestin-only methods, particularly LARCs, or long-acting reversible contraceptives, in both the control of bleeding and the prevention of pregnancy. These methods offer a reliable option for women who need long-term contraception with minimal daily compliance.

Complexities in the relationship combined with oral contraceptives (COCs) and anticonvulsant medications, particularly lamotrigine (LTG), present challenges for women with epilepsy (WWE). Recently, an interaction between these was researched by Rauchenzauner et al. [4], who showed that progestins, especially drospirenone and levonorgestrel, significantly lower LTG serum concentrations during active pill use, thereby increasing seizure risks. On the other hand, it did not affect progestin levels, thus suggesting that contraceptive efficacy is not affected. These findings indicate a need for cautious progestin selection in WWE to maintain therapeutic levels of LTG while ensuring effective contraception.

Nevertheless, the search for progestins has continued, and most of the newer compounds have fewer side effects, mostly without losing their efficacies. García-Sáenz et al. [1] drew attention to some new developments, including the anti-androgenic features of new progestins like drospirenone, which can reduce blood pressure, lower low-density lipoprotein (LDL) levels, and raise high-density lipoprotein (HDL) levels. Besides being safe during lactation, progestins are safe in the early postpartum period with no potential impact on milk composition or infant health. This mirrors an increasing tendency to tailor contraceptive options to individual needs and minimise risks.

5. *Mechanisms of progestin actions and progestin-specific activity via progesterone receptors:* Progestins exert a central and peripheral inhibitory action on pregnancy. García-Sáenz et al. [1] explained that the dual action of progestins involves central inhibition of gonadotropin release from the pituitary, resulting in no ovulation, and peripheral action on cervical mucus and the endometrium.

   The regulation of smooth muscle contraction is critical for tubal peristalsis and cervical mucus production, playing a vital role in reproductive health and contraception. Smooth muscle in the fallopian tubes facilitates the transport of the ovum toward the uterus through peristaltic movements, regulated by neural, hormonal, and paracrine signals [55]. Epithelial cells lining the tubes secrete factors like prostaglandins, which enhance smooth muscle contractility by increasing calcium influx into the cells [55]. This contraction mechanism involves complex biophysical processes, including changes in membrane potential and calcium channel activity [56]. In the cervix, cervical mucus varies in viscosity and composition throughout the menstrual cycle, influenced by hormonal changes and smooth muscle contractions. During ovulation, mucus becomes more fluid to allow sperm passage, while it thickens during non-fertile phases to create a barrier [55, 56].

   The interplay between smooth muscle contractions and cervical mucus is essential for creating a supportive environment for sperm during the fertile window. However, thickening of the cervical mucus and suppression of endometrial proliferation by progestins result in the inability of sperm to penetrate and an altered intrauterine environment that does not allow implantation [1]. In particular, drospirenone is not only a contraceptive but also possesses certain other features, including anti-androgenic and anti-mineralocorticoid effects, making this compound more attractive for many patients with specific health needs [1]. Progestins are a class of drugs with very diverse pharmacological profiles, especially when taken against the PR-A. Hence, Cartwright et al. [20] examined how progestins used in contraception and menopausal hormone therapy (MHT) differ in their efficacy and potency, depending on PR-A density. They identified that certain progestins, such as medroxyprogesterone acetate, norethisterone, and drospirenone, have distinct agonist properties dependent on the level of receptor expression. This might be interpreted as a receptor-specific activity indicating different contraceptive solutions tailored to differential tissue receptor density and function.

6. *Pharmacokinetics and metabolism of progestin use in contraception:* the pharmacokinetic profile, absorption, metabolism, and clearance of progestin can have a significant impact on its efficacy and side effects. Bick et al. [18] reviewed studies on the metabolism and serum concentrations of progestins used in contraception; they were recognised with remarkable individual women variability across studies. Differences in intrinsic characteristics between participants, plus non-standardised methodologies, complicate our understanding of progestin behaviour. Gaps in research studies further create the demand for more harmonious approaches regarding the study of progestins, especially regarding cardiovascular risk and susceptibility to cancers.

7. *Risk of blood clot to drospirenone-containing contraception:* Drospirenone-containing contraceptives have garnered attention for their hormonal regulation benefits, but concerns persist about their association with blood clot risk, particularly deep vein thrombosis (DVT). Research by Stalas et al. [57] points to a notably higher risk of DVT in users of drospirenone/ethinyl estradiol (DRSP/EE) compared to those taking norethindrone/ethinyl estradiol (NET/EE). The increased risk was observed across all age groups, with a more pronounced effect in women over 40. Additionally, a significant interaction between DRSP/EE and prednisone was identified, with concurrent use leading to a substantially elevated DVT risk. However, Foidart et al. [58] present newer formulations of drospirenone-containing contraceptives combined with estetrol, which demonstrate a reduced effect on blood clotting mechanisms compared to those with ethinylestradiol. This estetrol-drospirenone combination also offers a more predictable bleeding pattern and shows minimal impact on hemostatic parameters, suggesting it could pose a lower risk of blood clots. The addition of estetrol may thus reduce the thrombotic risks typically associated with DRSP/EE, making it a potentially safer option. In summary, while drospirenone-containing contraceptives, especially when combined with ethinylestradiol, show a higher risk for DVT compared to some other formulations, newer combinations with estetrol appear to lower that risk.

In summary, progestins play a significant role in contraception, from bleeding control through endometrial modulation, the management of ovarian reserve, high contraceptive efficacy, mechanisms of action, pharmacokinetics, and metabolism. However, with such challenges as irregular bleeding and the effect on ovarian reserve markers, critical analyses in the cited studies raise important issues for clinical consideration. It follows from integrating progestin into contraceptive management that these roles need to be weighed against each other to maximise benefits while minimising adverse effects.

2.2.5 Role of progestins in endometriosis

This section highlights and discusses the roles of progestins in endometriosis.

1. *Progestins and endometrial atrophy:* Progestins have been known to induce decidualisation and subsequent atrophy of endometrial tissue within the uterine

cavity and at ectopic sites in patients with endometriosis. This therapeutic effect arises from blocking the proliferative effect of oestrogen on the endometrium. García-Sáenz et al. [1] present evidence that progestins induce atrophy in hormonally dependent ectopic endometrial tissues, thereby causing a reduction in the painful and inflammatory manifestations of the disease. This capability of preventing the growth of endometrial lesions has made progestins an essential part of long-term therapy. The studies also pointed out that progestin growth inhibition acts in synergy with anovulation and suppression of ovarian steroidogenesis, which further reduces the cyclical exacerbation of endometrial lesions The evidence provided by Vercellini et al. [3] strongly supports the fact that progestins can induce endometrial atrophy. Their research underlines that progestins establish an anti-inflammatory and pro-apoptotic environment, significantly reducing endometrial tissue growth. This reduction in endometrial tissue is associated with a lesser chance of recurrence of symptoms, especially dysmenorrhea, which infers potential long-term therapeutic advantages.

2. *Progestins in pain management:* Endometriosis is often linked to persistent pelvic pain because of the body's inflammatory response and abnormal tissue growth. Progestins have been a crucial part of its medical treatment. In a study by Surrey [59], various progestins, including depot medroxyprogesterone acetate (DMPA), were found to lessen the intensity of pain associated with endometriosis effectively. Although there is a lack of large-scale, randomised studies, smaller trials have shown significant relief of symptoms, especially when progestins were administered through injections. Injectable progestins also help in reducing the recurrence of symptoms between doses.

   In line with Surrey [59], García-Sáenz et al. [1] emphasised that progestins hinder the growth of the endometrium and mitigate inflammatory reactions and oxidative stress, both of which are linked to the pain caused by endometriosis. Moreover, progestins decrease pro-inflammatory proteins like interleukins, thus providing further relief from the persistent pain related to this condition.

3. *Anti-inflammatory and anti-angiogenic effects of progestins:* Progestins are essential for reducing the inflammatory processes linked to endometriosis. According to García-Sáenz et al. [1], progestins hinder the release of important inflammatory substances like interleukin-6, interleukin-8, and monocyte chemotactic protein type 1. This anti-inflammatory effect has a greater implication in the alleviation of pain and lesions associated with endometriosis and, therefore, is of particular benefit for those patients in whom treatment with estrogens is contraindicated.

   Progestins also exhibit anti-angiogenic properties that inhibit the growth of new blood vessels supplying endometrial lesions. According to Vercellini et al. [3], these anti-angiogenic effects are related to the inhibition of nuclear factor kappa B (NF-κB), which is crucial in inflammation and neoangiogenesis. Progestin's prevention of neoangiogenesis reduces the proliferation of endometrial tissue and lowers the recurrence rates of the disease following surgical interventions.

4. *Progestins as fertility-sparing agents:* The role of progestins in fertility preservation is critical for women with endometriosis who desire pregnancy. The hormonal treatment aims to control disease progression while maintaining fertility

potential. Piatek et al. [60] and Yang et al. [61] both presented evidence of progestin-based therapies being effective in managing endometrial pathologies while allowing for successful pregnancies. In Yang et al. [61], a combination of hysteroscopic tumour resection followed by progestin therapy enabled women with early-stage endometrial cancer, who also suffered from endometriosis, to achieve complete remission and maintain their fertility. Similarly, Piatek et al. [60] highlighted that using progestins in patients with atypical endometrial hyperplasia resulted in significant rates of complete remission, allowing several patients to conceive successfully. The use of levonorgestrel-releasing intrauterine devices (IUDs) in this context was particularly effective, demonstrating higher remission rates than oral progestins. This underscores progestins' utility in both disease management and fertility preservation.

5. *Progestins and pregnancy complications in endometriosis:* Despite the benefits of using progestins to manage endometriosis and preserve fertility, they have been linked to certain pregnancy complications in women with the condition. According to Chiu and Wang [62], endometriosis increases the likelihood of negative outcomes for both the mother and the foetus, including conditions like pre-eclampsia, placental issues, and premature birth. However, these risks are typically related to the severity of the endometriosis rather than the progestin therapy itself. Therefore, while progestins can aid in achieving pregnancy for women with endometriosis, careful monitoring during pregnancy is crucial to reduce the chances of complications.

6. *Progesterone resistance in endometriosis:* Progesterone resistance plays a crucial role in understanding the fertility challenges faced by women with endometriosis, particularly in terms of embryo implantation and pregnancy success. Endometriosis is a chronic condition where tissue similar to the endometrium grows outside the uterus, often leading to infertility and pelvic pain. Studies by Alsbjerg et al. [63] and Racca et al. [64] provide valuable perspectives on how this resistance impacts endometrial receptivity and outcomes of embryo transfer. In women with endometriosis, progesterone resistance refers to the diminished response of the endometrial lining to progesterone, which is essential for preparing the uterus for embryo implantation. This resistance can disrupt the normal function of progesterone receptors, impacting gene expression necessary for a receptive endometrium, potentially leading to failed implantation. Alsbjerg et al. [63] explored this issue by examining serum progesterone levels during hormone replacement therapy frozen embryo transfer (HRT-FET) cycles in endometriosis patients. Their study revealed that patients with serum progesterone levels above 118 nmol/l had significantly higher live birth rates compared to those with lower levels, indicating that maintaining an optimal progesterone level is key to improving implantation and pregnancy outcomes. This finding suggests that sufficient progesterone supplementation may help overcome progesterone resistance in endometriosis patients.

   On the other hand, Racca et al. [64] explored the impact of endometriosis on endometrial receptivity in the context of IVF. They found that, despite the changes observed in endometrial tissue, endometriosis does not have a significant impact on receptivity or IVF success, particularly when frozen embryo transfers are performed during hormonally controlled cycles. This challenges the idea that progesterone resistance alone leads to lower implantation rates in women with endometriosis. Their findings also suggest that pre-treatment with hormonal therapy or surgical removal of endometriosis may not be necessary to enhance implantation rates in these patients.

These studies highlight that while progesterone resistance is a critical consideration in endometriosis-related infertility, it can be managed with appropriate hormonal therapy. Alsbjerg et al. (2023) identified an optimal progesterone threshold, offering practical advice for clinicians to improve reproductive outcomes through intensive progesterone support during the luteal phase. Meanwhile, Racca et al. [64] suggest that the negative impact of progesterone resistance on endometrial receptivity may not be as severe as previously thought, especially in controlled IVF treatments.

In summary, progestins have a multistep role in treating endometriosis, including inducing atrophy of the endometrium, reducing pain, anti-inflammatory and anti-angiogenic effects, and preserving fertility in the affected women. This, however, calls for close clinical monitoring for possible pregnancy complications. Progestins have been popularly acknowledged as long-term controllers of the disease with adequately established fertility-preserving potential. However, more extensive research is still needed to improve treatment approaches and minimise risks. Therefore, further studies will be needed in the future that will compare the efficacy of different types of progestins and routes of administration for a better understanding of their applications in clinical guidance.

2.2.6 Role of progestin in hormone replacement therapy

The following highlights and discusses the role of progestin in hormone replacement therapy (HRT).

1. *Protection against endometrial hyperplasia:* Progestins play an essential role in HRT to minimise the risks of endometrial hyperplasia and cancer associated with the use of unopposed oestrogen in postmenopausal women who have intact uteri. Lobo [65] emphasises that progestins should be an integral part of HRT modalities in such patients; further, he proposes using low doses of progestin, which block cell proliferation, thereby offering protection against cancer while exerting a minimum negative impact on therapeutic benefits. Similarly, García-Sáenz et al. [1] discuss progestins' role in protecting the endometrium and recommend that their potency and duration of use be individualised depending on needs but in such a way as to maximise efficacy while minimising adverse effects. Both sources stress the importance of a progestin dosage and type tailored to avoid hyperplasia with no additional complications.

2. *Bone health and osteoporosis prevention:* Progestins also play a role in maintaining bone health among postmenopausal women. According to Lobo [65], continuous therapy with oestrogen and progestin can enhance bone mineral density in women suffering from osteoporosis. This is important because it is quite well-documented that the lower levels of oestrogen after menopause contribute to the loss of bones. A combination of estradiol and Drospirenone (DRSP) was also noted by Vitale et al. [66] to improve vascular function and reduce arterial stiffness in postmenopausal women, indirectly positively influencing bone health. In both cited reports, the contribution of progestins to the maintenance of bone

health is underlined: the right balance between oestrogen and progestin optimises their combined positive action in skeletal health.

3. *Cardiovascular and metabolic impacts:* Progestins have been associated with controversial cardiovascular effects. According to Lobo [65], some progestins blunt the favourable effect of oestrogen by lowering HDL cholesterol and affecting arterial tone. This suggests that judicious selection and use of progestins are necessary to avoid the weakening of the favourable cardiovascular effects of oestrogen. On the other hand, the experiment by Vitale et al. [66] showed that Drospirenone was given along with estradiol, which resulted in favourable cardiovascular effects due to blood pressure reductions and improved endothelial function. This suggests that a progestin with good metabolic properties, such as Drospirenone, should be selected to minimise the risk of cardiovascular disease during HRT. Similarly, García-Sáenz et al. [1] insist on the balance between type and dosage of progestin to minimise adverse effects on the cardiovascular side but ensure therapeutic benefits.

4. *Breast cancer risk:* The link between progestins and breast cancer risk remains controversial. Africander and Toit [67] caution against assuming that all progestins increase breast cancer risk, pointing out that the effects of different progestins on breast tissue can vary significantly. They argue that more research is needed to distinguish between the actions of various progestins to avoid blanket assumptions about their risks. Similarly, Vogel [68] discusses the complex relationship between HRT and breast cancer risk, noting that progestins play a role in this association, but their impact depends on the specific type and the individual's hormonal background. Both sources stress the importance of personalising HRT to account for progestin-specific risks, particularly concerning breast cancer.

In summary, progestins play a multifaceted role in hormone replacement therapy (HRT), impacting aspects such as endometrial protection, bone health, and cardiovascular function. Lobo [65] emphasises the significance of selecting the right type and dosage of progestin to minimise risks while maintaining the advantages of HRT. García-Sáenz et al. [1] support this by highlighting the necessity of adjusting progestin treatment based on its potency and individual patient needs. However, the cardiovascular effects of progestins are still debated, with Lobo [65] urging caution due to potential negative impacts, while Vitale et al. [66] present evidence that Drospirenone may improve cardiovascular outcomes when used with Estradiol. This suggests that the choice of progestin should be personalised to each patient's health profile. Regarding breast cancer risk, Africander and Toit [67] and Vogel [68] emphasise that not all progestins pose the same level of risk, and it is essential to differentiate between their effects. These findings point to the need for a tailored approach in HRT, where the type of progestin is selected based on individual health factors and risk profiles rather than broad generalisations. This critical understanding ensures that HRT can be optimised for each woman, balancing benefits with minimised risks.

2.2.7 Role of progestin in assisted reproductive techniques

In this section, different themes are highlighted, and supporting literature is combined to present the roles of progestin in Assisted Reproductive Techniques in a well-organised critical discussion.

1. *Progestins and suppression of ovulation in IVF cycles:* Progestins have been recognised to suppress ovulation for IVF treatments and permit a "freeze-all" strategy where embryos are stored for transfer later. A study from Evans et al. [69] showed that while using progestin in fresh IVF cycles may not be the most cost-effective option, it does provide a financial advantage in planned "freeze-only" cycles. This is through the reduction of fresh embryo transfers and better endometrium receptivity in subsequent cycles.

2. *Progestin-primed ovarian stimulation (PPOS) and GnRH antagonist protocol in poor responders (POR):* In one recent study, the incidence of premature LH surges and oocyte retrieval outcomes were compared in women undergoing COS with either PPOS or a GnRH antagonist protocol [70]. The risk of premature LH surges was significantly lower in the former group (5.6% versus 16.9%). However, comparing oocyte retrieval rates and the number of oocytes retrieved did not differ significantly between groups. The authors postulated that PPOS is useful for cryopreservation but is not a full replacement in IVF cycles for GnRH antagonist protocols.

3. *Progestin and reversal of progestin resistance in endometrial cancer:* The microenvironment created by in vitro fertilisation can potentially overcome one of the most frequent obstacles to conservative management of endometrial cancers, namely progestin resistance. Sun et al. [71] demonstrated that fluid from the IVF-generated embryo reversed progestin resistance in endometrial cancer stem cells. This occurred through the downregulation of key stemness genes via epigenetic modulation, thus enabling the differentiation of CSCs and enhancing their sensitivity to the progestin treatment.

4. *Progestin use in exotic animal reproduction:* The role of progestin in augmenting the ovarian response to ART in humans are parallels among animal populations. For instance, one investigation in cheetahs showed that pre-administration with oral progestin augmented the ovarian response after exogenous gonadotropin stimulation [72]. The above study findings for genetic management in this threatened species are relevant because they allowed the conclusion that oral progestin pre-medication could induce a more favourable ovarian response, as evidenced by increased levels of estradiol and decreased levels of glucocorticoids.

5. *Oral progestin and suppression of ovarian activity in cats:* Stewart et al. [73] investigated oral progestin to suppress ovarian activity in domestic cats. They identified that oral progestin suppressed follicular activity within a short time, which was succeeded by a restoration of ovarian activity within a very short period after cessation of treatment. This study illustrates the potential of progestin priming as a strategy to improve the success rate of ovulation induction for ART in felids.

6. *Progestins roles in GnRH analogues:* Alexandru et al. [74], through an extensive review and analysis, compared the effectiveness of progestins with that of GnRH analogues for pituitary suppression in ovarian stimulation of ART. Progestins seem equally effective as GnRH antagonists in preventing premature ovulation and result in significantly higher live birth or ongoing pregnancy rates per embryo transfer compared with the short GnRH agonist protocol. However, the progestin-stimulated cycles did require extended stimulation with more gonadotropins, though clinically these differences were regarded not significant.

7. *Flexible progestin-primed ovarian stimulation (fPPOS) and GnRH antagonist protocol:* Yildiz et al. [75] compared the fPPOS protocol with the GnRH antagonist protocol in oocyte donors. They noticed that the fPPOS protocol yielded higher numbers of cumulus-oocyte complexes and metaphase II oocytes than the cycles from GnRH antagonist administration. Nonetheless, pregnancy rates were no different in recipients of fresh oocytes originating from either protocol, indicating that fPPOS is a comparable alternative to prevent premature ovulation without affecting oocyte quality.

8. *Progestin serves as an economical approach in ART:* Progestins have emerged as the most attractive option in ovarian stimulation in assisted reproductive technology due to their cost and ease of administration. Capuzzo and La Marca [76] reported that progestins can be used to prevent ovulation without compromising endometrial receptivity after the improvements in cryopreservation techniques. Moreover, they discussed that progestin-primed stimulation could be an excellent option when a freeze-all strategy could be foreseen in hyper-responders, fertility preservation, and oocyte donors.

Incorporating progestins into ART protocols has several advantages, including suppressing premature ovulation and improving ovarian response in both human and animal studies. While further large-scale research is necessary to confirm these conclusions, existing evidence suggests that progestin-primed stimulation is a successful, safe, and potentially more economical alternative to traditional GnRH antagonist protocols.

3. Conclusion

Progestins are synthetic versions of natural progesterone and consist of progestins such as medroxyprogesterone acetate and norethindrone. These drugs are necessary for reproduction. They control menstruation flow by maintaining consistent levels in the endometrial lining and averting menstrual disorders. They act to offset the effects of oestrogen to prevent early ovulation. In specific assisted reproductive techniques, hormonal medications are employed to control the timing of ovulation and improve the conditions for egg retrieval or embryo transfer. Progestins are involved in maintaining the uterine lining, preventing early uterine contractions, and aiding in the embryo's implantation and the fetus's growth during pregnancy. Conversely, progestin-based contraceptives function by preventing ovulation, thickening cervical mucus, and modifying the endometrial lining to deter fertilisation and implantation. While some of the assisted reproduction technologies have utilised progestins in controlling the time of ovulation and optimisation of conditions for either egg retrieval or embryo transfer. Progestins are crucial during pregnancy, promoting the maintenance of the uterus lining, preventing premature uterine contractions, the implantation of the embryo, and fetal growth. Progestins also play an important role in HRT by balancing hormones, relieving symptoms of menopause, and preventing endometrial hyperplasia when administered with estrogens. They are also useful in treating endometriosis by causing atrophy of the endometrial tissue and less growth of oestrogen-driven lesions, hence alleviating symptoms to a great degree. In ART, progestins are useful in controlled ovarian stimulation and enhancement of endometrial receptivity, thus improving the outcomes of fertility procedures. They also benefit in the treatment of endometriosis through atrophy of the endometrial tissue and less growth of oestrogen-driven lesions, hence alleviating symptoms to a great degree. The diversified profile of progestins in action underlines their importance for managing reproductive health, enhancing fertility, ensuring effective contraception, and also the treatment of endometriosis and menopausal symptoms. Further research into progestins is needed to optimise their therapeutic benefits and overcome some of the challenges in reproductive medicine and hormonal management. The chapter will contribute to knowledge, inform relevant policies, and improve medical practices in reproductive medicine to realise effective management strategies and better overall care.

Acknowledgements

The authors of this book chapter acknowledge the following persons, my lovely wife Blessing Onyeso, Onuoha Rejoice, Ekaba Samson Gift, and host of others for their input toward the development of this chapter.

Conflict of interest

The authors have no conflict of interest to declare.

Notes/thanks/other declarations

Thank you IntechOpen, for offering us the opportunity to be involved in developing this book chapter. We look forward to working with you in the future.

Author details

Godspower Onyeso[1*], Japheth David[2], Michael Egwu[3] and Menizibeya Welcome[4]

1 Department of Human Physiology, Faculty of Basic Medical Sciences, College of Medical Sciences, Rivers State University, Port-Harcourt, Nigeria

2 Department of Preventive and Social Medicine, Faculty of Clinical Sciences, University of Port-Harcourt, Port-Harcourt, Nigeria

3 Nisa Premier Hospital, Abuja, Nigeria

4 Department of Human Physiology, Faculty of Basic Medical Sciences, College of Health Sciences, Nile University of Nigeria, FCT – Abuja, Nigeria

*Address all correspondence to: godspower.onyeso@ust.edu.ng

References

[1] García-Sáenz M, Ibarra-Salce R, Pozos-Varela FJ, Mena-Ureta TS, Flores-Villagómez S, Ferreira-Hermosillo A. Understanding progestins: From basics to clinical applicability. Journal of Clinical Medicine. 2023;**12**(10):3388. DOI: 10.3390/jcm12103388

[2] Laurora I, Henrie B, Guillard H, Bradford R, Sober S, Glasier A. Evaluation of adherence to a daily progestin-only pill in a simulated over-the-counter setting. Contraception. 2024;**133**:110388. DOI: 10.1016/j.contraception.2024.110388

[3] Vercellini P, Buggio L, Berlanda N, Barbara G, Somigliana E, Bosari S. Estrogen-progestins and progestins for the management of endometriosis. Fertility and Sterility. 2016;**106**:1552-1571. DOI: 10.1016/j.fertnstert.2016.10.022

[4] Rauchenzauner M, Deichmann S, Pittschieler S, Bergmann M, Prieschl M, Unterberger I, et al. Bidirectional interaction between oral contraception and lamotrigine in women with epilepsy – Role of progestins. Seizure. 2020;**74**:89-92. DOI: 10.1016/j.seizure.2019.11.011

[5] Song JY, Fraser IS. Effects of progestogens on human endometrium. Obstetrical & Gynaecological survey. 1995;**50**(5):385-394. DOI: 10.1097/00006254-199505000-00026

[6] Cable JK, Grider MH. Physiology, progesterone. In: StatPearls. Treasure Island, FL: StatPearls Publishing; 2023. pp. 1-15. Available from: https://www.ncbi.nlm.nih. gov/books/NBK558960/ [Accessed: September 10, 2024]

[7] Elliott-Sale KJ, Flood TR, Arent SM. Effect of menstrual cycle and contraceptive pill phase on aspects of exercise physiology and athletic performance in female athletes: Protocol for the Feminae international multisite innovative project. BMJ Open Sport & Exercise Medicine. 2023;**9**(1):e001814. DOI: 10.1136/bmjsem-2023-001814

[8] Malik MA, Nadeem MS. Molecular mechanism of action of estrogens, progestins, and androgens. How Synthetic Drugs Work. 2023;**1**:123-159. DOI: 10.1016/B978-0-323-99855-0.00006-3

[9] Edwards M, Can AS. Progestins. In: StatPearls. Treasure Island, FL: StatPearls Publishing; 2024. pp. 1-10. Available from: https:// www.ncbi.nlm.nih.gov/books/ NBK563211/ [Accessed: September 10, 2024]

[10] Malhotra A, Singh R, Acharya PC, Bansal R. Hormones and antihormones in cancer chemotherapy. In: Acharya PC, Kurosu M, editors. Medicinal Chemistry of Chemotherapeutic Agents. Cambridge, MA: Academic Press; 2023. pp. 589-613. DOI: 10.1016/B978-0-323-90575-6.00004-1

[11] Sitruk-Ware R. New progestagens for contraceptive use. Human Reproduction Update. 2006;**12**(2):169-178. DOI: 10.1093/humupd/dmi046

[12] Chen M, Penning TM. 5β-reduced steroids and human Δ(4)-3-ketosteroid 5β-reductase (AKR1D1). Steroids. 2014;**83**:17-26. DOI: 10.1016/j.steroids.2014.01.013

[13] Stanczyk FZ, Hapgood JP, Winer S, Mishell DR Jr. Progestogens used in postmenopausal hormone therapy: Differences in their pharmacological properties, intracellular actions, and

clinical effects. Endocrine Reviews. 2013;**34**(2):171-208. DOI: 10.1210/er.2012-1008

[14] Stanczyk F. All progestins are not created equal. Steroids. 2003;**68**:879-890. DOI: 10.1016/j.steroids.2003.08.003

[15] Ferrero S. Progesterone and progestin mimics. In: Wexler P, editor. Encyclopedia of Toxicology. 4th ed. Cambridge, MA: Academic Press; 2024. pp. 903-909. DOI: 10.1016/B978-0-12-824315-2.01139-8

[16] Lessey BA, Young SL. Structure, function, and evaluation of the female reproductive tract. In: Strauss JF, Barbieri RL, editors. Yen and Jaffe's Reproductive Endocrinology. 8th ed. Philadelphia, PA: Elsevier; 2019. pp. 206-247.e13. DOI: 10.1016/B978-0-323-47912-7.00009-3

[17] Motwani R, Krishna H. Ovulation. In: Shackelford TK, editor. Encyclopedia of Sexual Psychology and Behavior. Cham: Springer; 2024. pp. 1-6. DOI: 10.1007/978-3-031-08956-5_302-1

[18] Bick AJ, Louw-du Toit R, Skosana SB, Africander D, Hapgood JP. Pharmacokinetics, metabolism and serum concentrations of progestins used in contraception. Pharmacology & Therapeutics. 2021;**222**:107789. DOI: 10.1016/j.pharmthera.2020.107789

[19] Pascual ZN, Langaker MD. Physiology, pregnancy. In: StatPearls [Internet]. Treasure Island, FL: StatPearls Publishing; 2023. Available from: https://www.ncbi.nlm.nih. gov/books/NBK559304/ [Accessed: September 10, 2024]

[20] Cartwright M, Louw-du Toit R, Africander D. The transcriptional activity of progestins used in contraception and menopausal hormone therapy via progesterone receptor A is dependent on the density of the receptor. Biochemical and Biophysical Research Communications. 2023;**639**:70-76. DOI: 10.1016/j.bbrc.2022.11.077

[21] Jain R, Muralidhar S. Contraceptive methods: Needs, options and utilization. Journal of Obstetrics and Gynaecology of India. 2011;**61**(6):626-634. DOI: 10.1007/s13224-011-0107-7

[22] Moura APC, Novis MI, Demarchi GTS, Fernandes LM, D'Ippolito G, Torres US, et al. Pelvic hemorrhagic lesions in women: MRI findings and differential diagnosis. Clinical Imaging. 2020;**60**(1):16-25. DOI: 10.1016/j.clinimag.2019.12.008

[23] Saunders PTK, Horne AW. Endometriosis: Etiology, pathobiology, and therapeutic prospects. Cell. 2021;**184**(11):2807-2824. DOI: 10.1016/j.cell.2021.04.041

[24] Harper-Harrison G, Carlson K, Shanahan MM. Hormone replacement therapy. In: StatPearls. StatPearls Publishing; 2024. Available from: https://www.ncbi.nlm.nih.gov/books/NBK493191/ [Accessed: September 10, 2024]

[25] Graham ME, Jelin A, Hoon AH Jr, Wilms Floet AM, Levey E, Graham EM. Assisted reproductive technology: Short- and long-term outcomes. Developmental Medicine and Child Neurology. 2023;**65**(1):38-49. DOI: 10.1111/dmcn.15332

[26] Berga SL, Johnston-MacAnanny EB. Physiology of the menstrual cycle. In: Bieber EJ, Sanfilippo JS, Horowitz IR, Shafi MI, editors. Clinical Gynecology. Cambridge: Cambridge University Press; 2015. pp. 972-984

[27] Schatz F, Krikun G, Caze R, Rahman M, Lockwood CJ.

Progestin-regulated expression of tissue factor in decidual cells: Implications in endometrial hemostasis, menstruation and angiogenesis. Steroids. 2003;**68**(10-13):849-860. DOI: 10.1016/S0039-128X(03)00139-9

[28] Avila-Varela DS, Hidalgo-Lopez E, Dagnino PC, Del Agua E, Deco G, Pletzer B, et al. Whole-brain dynamics across the menstrual cycle: The role of hormonal fluctuations and age in healthy women. Npj Women's Health. 2024;**2**(1):1-9. DOI: 10.1038/s44294-024-00012-4

[29] Grindlay K, Obedin-Maliver J, Ragosta S, Hastings J, Lunn MR, Flentje A, et al. Interest in over-the-counter progestin-only pills among transgender, nonbinary, and gender-expansive individuals in the United States. American Journal of Obstetrics and Gynecology. 2024;**230**(6):657.e1-657.e17. DOI: 10.1016/j.ajog.2024.02.006

[30] Bonnema J, Dalebout JA. The abuse of high dose estrogen/progestin combination drugs in delay of menstruation: The assumptions and practices of doctors, midwives and pharmacists in a Peruvian city. Social Science & Medicine. 1992;**34**(3):281-289. DOI: 10.1016/0277-9536(92)90270-Z

[31] Pelican KM, Wildt DE, Ottinger MA, Howard J. Priming with progestin, but not GnRH antagonist, induces a consistent endocrine response to exogenous gonadotropins in induced and spontaneously ovulating cats. Domestic Animal Endocrinology. 2008;**34**(2):160-175. DOI: 10.1016/j.domaniend.2007.01.002

[32] Storer WA, Thompson DL, Gilley RM, Burns PJ. Evaluation of injectable sustained release progestin formulations for suppression of estrus and ovulation in mares. Journal of Equine Veterinary Science. 2009;**29**(1):33-36. DOI: 10.1016/j.jevs.2008.11.007

[33] Endrikat J, Gerlinger C, Richard S, Rosenbaum P, Düsterberg B. Ovulation inhibition doses of progestins: A systematic review of the available literature and of marketed preparations worldwide. Contraception. 2011;**84**(6):549-557. DOI: 10.1016/j.contraception.2011.04.009

[34] La Marca A, Capuzzo M. Use of progestins to inhibit spontaneous ovulation during ovarian stimulation: The beginning of a new era? Reproductive BioMedicine Online. 2019;**39**(2):321-331. DOI: 10.1016/j.rbmo.2019.03.212

[35] Cosentino IO, Balaro MFA, Leal FSC, Bade ALC, Brandão FZ. Ovarian activity in dairy Saanen goats subjected to a short-term ovulation induction protocol and a single injection of lecirelin (GnRH analog) given 28 h or 34 h after progestin pre-treatment. Small Ruminant Research. 2020;**191**:106214. DOI: 10.1016/j.smallrumres.2020.106214

[36] Xie Y, Guo W, Shen X, Yu W, Kuang Y, Chen Q, et al. A delayed ovulation of progestin-primed ovarian stimulation (PPOS) by downregulating the LHCGR/PGR pathway. IScience. 2023;**26**(8):107357. DOI: 10.1016/j.isci.2023.107357

[37] Takahashi T, Ogiwara K. Signal pathway of LH-induced expression of nuclear progestin receptor in vertebrate ovulation. General and Comparative Endocrinology. 2022;**321-322**:114025. DOI: 10.1016/j.ygcen.2022.114025

[38] Chen ZQ, Ai A, Zhang Y, Li H, Wang JY, Wang L, et al. A randomized controlled trial to compare the live birth rate of the first frozen embryo transfer following the progestin-primed ovarian

stimulation protocol vs. the antagonist protocol in women with an anticipated high ovarian response. Fertility and Sterility. 2024;**121**(6):937-945. DOI: 10.1016/j.fertnstert.2024.01.027

[39] Goodman LR, Smith LP, Purcell S, Williams CD. Progestin ovulation suppression in oocyte cryopreservation cycles reduces financial and logistical burden without compromising yield. Fertility and Sterility. 2024;**122**(1):e31. DOI: 10.1016/j.fertnstert.2024.05.053

[40] Wu X, Liu D, Chen S, Hong W, Zhu Y. Impaired oocyte maturation and ovulation in membrane progestin receptor (mPR) knockouts in zebrafish. Molecular and Cellular Endocrinology. 2020;**511**:110856. DOI: 10.1016/j.mce.2020.110856

[41] Cai R, Zheng B, Lin Q, Deng J, Zeng X, Lin W, et al. A meta-analysis of the efficacy of progestin-primed ovarian stimulation with medroxyprogesterone acetate in ovulation induction in poor ovarian responders. Journal of Gynecology Obstetrics and Human Reproduction. 2021;**50**(7):102049. DOI: 10.1016/j.jogoh.2020.102049

[42] Pai AHY, Sung YJ, Li CJ, Lin CY, Chang CL. Progestin primed ovarian stimulation (PPOS) protocol yields lower euploidy rate in older patients undergoing IVF. Reproductive Biology and Endocrinology. 2023;**21**:72. DOI: 10.1186/s12958-023-01124-3

[43] Guillard H, Laurora I, Sober S, Karapet A, Brass EP, Glasier A. Modeling the potential benefit of an over-the-counter progestin-only pill in preventing unintended pregnancies in the U.S. Contraception. 2023;**117**:7-12. DOI: 10.1016/j.contraception.2022.10.006

[44] Wollum A, Trussell J, Grossman D, Grindlay K. Modeling the impacts of price of an over-the-counter progestin-only pill on use and unintended pregnancy among U.S. women. Women's Health Issues. 2020;**30**(3):153-160. DOI: 10.1016/j.whi.2020.01.003

[45] Callahan R, Yacobson I, Halpern V, Nanda K. Ectopic pregnancy with use of progestin-only injectables and contraceptive implants: A systematic review. Contraception. 2015;**92**(6):514-522. DOI: 10.1016/j.contraception.2015.08.016

[46] Byrns MC. Regulation of progesterone signalling during pregnancy: Implications for the use of progestins for the prevention of preterm birth. The Journal of Steroid Biochemistry and Molecular Biology. 2014;**139**:173-181. DOI: 10.1016/j.jsbmb.2013.01.015

[47] Boelig RC, Della Corte L, Ashoush S, McKenna D, Saccone G, Rajaram S, et al. Oral progesterone for the prevention of recurrent preterm birth: Systematic review and meta-analysis. American Journal of Obstetrics & Gynecology MFM. 2019;**1**(1):50-62. DOI: 10.1016/j.ajogmf.2019.03.001

[48] Katalinic A, Shulman LP, Strauss JF, Garcia-Velasco JA, Van den Anker JN. A critical appraisal of safety data on dydrogesterone for the support of early pregnancy: A scoping review and meta-analysis. Reproductive BioMedicine Online. 2022;**45**(2):365-373. DOI: 10.1016/j.rbmo.2022.03.032

[49] Shikichi M, Iwata K, Ito K, Miyakoshi D, Murase H, Sato F, et al. Abnormal pregnancies associated with deviation in progestin and estrogen profiles in late pregnant mares: A diagnostic aid. Theriogenology. 2017;**98**:75-81. DOI: 10.1016/j.theriogenology.2017.04.024

[50] Akay MA, Yıldız GE. Impact of gestational and parental factors and maternal intake of progesterone on the development of hypospadias: A retrospective case–control study. Taiwanese Journal of Obstetrics and Gynecology. 2021;**60**(5):894-898. DOI: 10.1016/j.tjog.2021.08.001

[51] Shoupe D. The progestin revolution: Progestins are arising as the dominant players in the tight interlink between contraceptives and bleeding control. Contraception and Reproductive Medicine. 2021;**6**:3. DOI: 10.1186/s40834-020-00142-5

[52] Edelman A, Boniface E, Schrote K, Messerle-Forbes M, O'Donnell A, Jensen JT, et al. Treatment of unfavorable bleeding patterns in contraceptive implant users: A randomized clinical trial of curcumin. American Journal of Obstetrics and Gynecology. 2023;**229**(2):145.e1-145.e9. DOI: 10.1016/j.ajog.2023.04.028

[53] Mandelbaum RS, Ciccone MA, Nusbaum DJ, Khoshchehreh M, Matsuo K. Progestin therapy for obese women with complex atypical hyperplasia: Levonorgestrel-releasing intrauterine device vs systemic therapy. American Journal of Obstetrics and Gynecology. 2020;**223**(1):103.e1-103.e13. DOI: 10.1016/j.ajog.2019.12.273

[54] Hariton E, Shirazi TN, Douglas NC, Hershlag A, Briggs SF. Anti-Müllerian hormone levels among contraceptive users: Evidence from a cross-sectional cohort of 27,125 individuals. American Journal of Obstetrics and Gynecology. 2021;**225**(5):515.e1-515.e10. DOI: 10.1016/j.ajog.2021.06.052

[55] Ruan YC, Zhou W, Chan HC. Regulation of smooth muscle contraction by the epithelium: Role of prostaglandins. Physiology (Bethesda). 2011;**26**(3):156-170. DOI: 10.1152/physiol.00036.2010

[56] Mahapatra C, Kumar R. Biophysical mechanisms of vaginal smooth muscle contraction: The role of the membrane potential and ion channels. Pathophysiology. 2024;**31**(2):225-243. DOI: 10.3390/pathophysiology31020018

[57] Stalas J, Morris R, Bu K, Von Bargen K, Largmann R, Sanford K, et al. Comparing the risk of deep vein thrombosis of two combined oral contraceptives: Norethindrone/ethinyl estradiol and drospirenone/ethinyl estradiol. Heliyon. 2024;**10**(5):e26462. DOI: 10.1016/j.heliyon.2024.e26462

[58] Foidart JM, Gemzell-Danielsson K, Kubba A, Douxfils J, Creinin MD, Gaspard U. The benefits of estetrol addition to drospirenone for contraception. AJOG Global Reports. 2023;**3**(4):100266. DOI: 10.1016/j.xagr.2023.100266

[59] Surrey ES. The role of progestins in treating the pain of endometriosis. Journal of Minimally Invasive Gynecology. 2006;**13**(6):528-534. DOI: 10.1016/j.jmig.2006.06.008

[60] Piatek S, Michalski W, Sobiczewski P, Bidzinski M, Szewczyk G. The results of different fertility-sparing treatment modalities and obstetric outcomes in patients with early endometrial cancer and atypical endometrial hyperplasia: Case series of 30 patients and systematic review. European Journal of Obstetrics &Gynecology and Reproductive Biology. 2021;**263**:139-147. DOI: 10.1016/j.ejogrb.2021.06.007

[61] Yang H, Liu J, Liu F. Fertility-preserving treatment of stage IA, well-differentiated endometrial carcinoma in young women with hysteroscopic resection and high-dose progesterone therapy. Taiwanese Journal of Obstetrics

and Gynecology. 2019;**58**(1):90-93. DOI: 10.1016/j.tjog.2018.11.017

[62] Chiu K, Wang I. Endometriosis, pregnancy and delivery complications: Evidence from the US nationwide inpatient sample 2005-2018. Taiwanese Journal of Obstetrics and Gynecology. 2024;**63**(3):350-356. DOI: 10.1016/j.tjog.2023.06.005

[63] Alsbjerg B, Kesmodel US, Humaidan P. Endometriosis patients benefit from high serum progesterone in hormone replacement therapy–frozen embryo transfer cycles: A cohort study. Reproductive BioMedicine Online. 2023;**46**(1):92-98. DOI: 10.1016/j.rbmo.2022.09.005

[64] Racca A, Bernabeu A, Bernabeu R, Ferrero S. Endometrial receptivity in women with endometriosis. Best Practice & Research Clinical Obstetrics & Gynaecology. 2024;**92**:102438. DOI: 10.1016/j.bpobgyn.2023.102438

[65] Lobo RA. The role of progestins in hormone replacement therapy. American Journal of Obstetrics and Gynecology. 1992;**166**(6):1997-2004. DOI: 10.1016/0002-9378(92)91401-U

[66] Vitale C, Mammi C, Gambacciani M, Russo N, Spoletini I, Fini M, et al. Effect of hormone replacement therapy with the anti-mineralocorticoid progestin Drospirenone compared to tibolone on endothelial function and central haemodynamics in post-menopausal women. International Journal of Cardiology. 2017;**227**:217-221. DOI: 10.1016/j.ijcard.2016.11.149

[67] Africander D, Toit RLD. Progestins in menopausal hormone therapy and breast cancer risk: The debate continues. Current Opinion in Endocrine and Metabolic Research. 2020;**15**:24-30. DOI: 10.1016/j.coemr.2020.10.001

[68] Vogel VG. Perils of progestins: Increased breast cancer risk associated with postmenopausal hormone replacement therapy. Breast Diseases: A Year Book Quarterly. 2008;**19**(2):123-126. DOI: 10.1016/S1043-321X(08)80076-8

[69] Evans MB, Parikh T, DeCherney AH, Csokmay JM, Healy MW, Hill MJ. Evaluation of the cost-effectiveness of ovulation suppression with progestins compared with GnRH analogs in assisted reproduction cycles. Reproductive BioMedicine Online. 2019;**38**(5):691-698. DOI: 10.1016/j.rbmo.2018.12.044

[70] Kao T, Hsieh Y, Yang I, Wu M, Chen M, Yang J, et al. Progestin-primed ovarian stimulation versus GnRH antagonist protocol in poor responders: Risk of premature LH surge and outcome of oocyte retrieval. Journal of the Formosan Medical Association. 2023;**122**(1):29-35. DOI: 10.1016/j.jfma.2022.08.023

[71] Sun D, Qin Z, Xu Y, Xiao Q, Xu Y, Bai M, et al. The IVF-generated human embryonic microenvironment reverses progestin resistance in endometrial cancer cells by inducing cancer stem cell differentiation. Cancer Letters. 2022;**526**:311-321. DOI: 10.1016/j.canlet.2021.11.003

[72] Thuwanut P, Brown JL, Comizzoli P, Crosier AE. Responsiveness of the cheetah (Acinonyx jubatus) ovary to exogenous gonadotropins after preemptive oral progestin treatment. Theriogenology. 2019;**138**:39-46. DOI: 10.1016/j.theriogenology.2019.07.001

[73] Stewart R, Pelican K, Brown J, Wildt D, Ottinger M, Howard J. Oral progestin induces rapid, reversible suppression of ovarian activity in the cat. General and Comparative Endocrinology.

2010;**166**(2):409-416. DOI: 10.1016/j.ygcen.2009.12.016

[74] Alexandru P, Cekic SG, Yildiz S, Turkgeldi E, Ata B. Progestins versus GnRH analogues for pituitary suppression during ovarian stimulation for assisted reproductive technology: A systematic review and meta-analysis. Reproductive BioMedicine Online. 2020;**40**(6):894-903. DOI: 10.1016/j.rbmo.2020.01.027

[75] Yildiz S, Turkgeldi E, Angun B, Eraslan A, Urman B, Ata B. Comparison of a novel flexible progestin primed ovarian stimulation protocol and the flexible gonadotropin-releasing hormone antagonist protocol for assisted reproductive technology. Fertility and Sterility. 2019;**112**(4):677-683. DOI: 10.1016/j.fertnstert.2019.06.009

[76] Capuzzo M, La Marca A. The use of progestins to prevent the LH surge in IVF cycles. In: Dahan MH, Fatemi HM, Polyzos NP, Garcia-Velasco JA, editors. Handbook of Current and Novel Protocols for the Treatment of Infertility. Cambridge, MA: Academic Press; 2024. pp. 179-188. DOI: 10.1016/B978-0-323-85687-4.00014-2

Section 3

Androgens

Chapter 5

Disorder-Related Sex Steroid Hormonal Production: Polycystic Ovarian Syndrome

I Gusti Agung Ngurah Agung Sentosa and Angel Benny Wisan

Abstract

Polycystic ovarian syndrome (PCOS) is a common gynaecological and endocrine illness that causes irregular menstruation, inadequate follicular development, interrupted ovulation, and decreased conception rates in women of reproductive age. The aetiology and available treatments for these symptoms are still restricted, although they can be controlled with the appropriate medicine and lifestyle changes. The two main characteristics of PCOS are elevated androgen levels (hyperandrogenism) and the luteinizing hormone/follicle-stimulating hormone (LH/FSH) ratio. The causes of androgen excess, synthesis, and androgen receptor (AR) signalling that mediate negative PCOS features are examined in this review, along with the role of adrenal-derived 11-oxygenated androgens in the pathogenesis of PCOS. It also offers treatment plans that specifically address hyperandrogenism in PCOS, emphasising how crucial it is to comprehend the processes involved in androgen synthesis, conversion, and metabolism in PCOS.

Keywords: hyperandrogen, insulin resistance, obesity, infertility, oligomenorrhea

1. Introduction

PCOS affects 8–13% of women, with diagnostic recommendations often unclear, leading to 70% misdiagnosis, highlighting the unclear genesis and aetiology of the condition [1–4]. Over the years, three diagnostic criteria have been developed for PCOS in women, with the Rotterdam 2003 criteria being the most widely used, though not universally accepted [5–7]. PCOS, an endocrine disorder, is characterised by three definitions: oligo-ovulatory infertility, hyperandrogenism, and polycystic ovarian morphology. The first definition was described by Stein and Leventhal in 1935. The classification was suggested by the National Institutes of Health/National Institute of Child Health and Human Development in 1990 [1, 3]. The Rotterdam classification includes oligoovulation, hyperandrogenism, and polycystic ovarian morphology. Previous PCOS consensual workshops focused on diagnosis and control [8–10].

The third PCOS consensus document outlines major aspects of PCOS, including knowledge gaps. The 2006 conference suggested parameters for PCOS diagnosis, including ovarian dysfunction, excess androgen production, and hyperandrogenism [3, 6]. However, these categories excluded certain conditions with similar symptoms. Four different phenotypic expressions have been identified: persistent anovulation and hyperandrogenism, hyperandrogenism and ultrasound-detected polycystic ovarian morphology, prolonged anovulation without hyperandrogenism, and hyperandrogenism combined with polycystic ovaries and chronic anovulations [8, 10–12].

PCOS diagnosis requires excluding other endocrine disorders like hyperprolactinaemia, thyroid disease, Non-classical Congenital Adrenal Hyperplasia (NCAH), Cushing's syndrome, hypogonadotropic hypogonadism, or androgen-producing tumours [3, 4]. Measurements of 17-hydroxyprogesterone levels, prolactin levels, and TSH levels can help differentiate between PCOS and other endocrine disorders. Cushing syndrome, characterised by obesity, hypertension, and amenorrhoea-like symptoms, can be distinguished from PCOS using dexamethasone suppression tests, 24-hour free urine cortisol or salivary cortisol tests [6–8]. Teenage women's diagnosis is based on biochemical and clinical indicators of hyperandrogenism with chronic oligomenorrhea [13].

2. Aetiology of PCOS

PCOS is a complex condition influenced by heritable and environmental factors [1]. The "two-hit" theory suggests a genetically predisposed factor develops after exposure to a postnatal stimulating factor, with insulin-resistant hyperinsulinism being the main postnatal factor [14, 15]. Another theory suggests that metabolic disorders like obesity and diabetes have evolutionary origins due to survival advantage, with insulin resistance contributing to these traits, possibly influencing the association of PCOS and 21-hydroxylase deficiency [1]. PCOS is a hereditary condition with varying degrees of dominant inheritance [4]. Over 70% of cases are inherited, with 50% of sisters being hyperandrogenic or amenorrhoeic [7]. About 25% of mothers are affected [16]. Postmenarchal symptoms, central obesity, and blood pressure increase, with 15 daughters meeting adult hyperandrogenic PCOS criteria [17].

A novel regulatory protein variant, DENND1A.V2, was discovered in 2014, explaining typical PCOS secretory abnormalities [4, 16]. The DENND1A isoform 1A, variant 2, has an extrapotent splice variant called V2, which mediates the PCOS steroidogenic anomaly in culture [11, 15]. 50% of PCOS families carry at least one of the 32 uncommon DENND1A mutations, supporting the theory that causal DENND1A variations occur in important genes [15–17]. A microRNA called miR-130b-3p, involved in gene expression regulation, has been linked to PCOS [11]. It suppresses luteinizing hormone receptor expression and interacts with insulin signalling *via* the Mitogen-activated protein kinase (MAPK) pathway [11, 16]. Forskolin stimulation activates steroidogenesis. 6.7% of PCOS patients with increased serum AMH levels have polymorphisms in the coding of anti-Müllerian hormone and AMH receptor, potentially due to inadequate inhibition of gatekeeper functions. This study suggests a primary folliculogenesis deficit may be the cause [16–18].

PCOS is often caused by congenital virilization, a method used to create models for experiments [17, 19]. This process reproduces reproductive and metabolic issues like obesity and insulin resistance in rhesus monkeys [19]. However, congenital virilization is unlikely to cause typical PCOS. Impaired prenatal nutrition, particularly foetal undernutrition, increases the risk of metabolic syndrome and cardiovascular disease [20, 21]. PCOS cases are primarily caused by normal birth weights, with epigenetic programming linking intrauterine disruptions to adult illness [4, 17].

Abnormal methylation of genes, aberrant miRNA expression, and differentially methylated sites in PCOS granulosa cells indicate epigenomic changes [17, 22]. PCOS and PCOS daughters have different DNA methylation levels. Prenatal androgen exposure causes transgenerational expression of genes in mouse oocytes and PCOS, while Tia1 cytotoxic granule-associated RNA binding protein-like 1 may play a role in androgen excess [23, 24].

Obesity exacerbates of PCOS symptoms in adolescents, with childhood obesity and PCOS predisposed by hereditary factors [22]. Pseudo-Cushing syndrome and pseudoacromegaly are rare diseases predicting PCOS in adolescents due to moderately severe insulin-resistant hyperinsulinism [24]. Reversible functional ovarian hyperandrogenism and PCOM are caused by virilization of sexually mature women [25, 26].

3. Pathophysiology of PCOS

A number of factors contribute to the complex pathophysiology of PCOS, including insulin resistance, fat accumulation, particularly in the abdominal area, hyperandrogenism, and hypothalamic-pituitary-ovarian axis dysfunction, which are caused by abnormalities in steroidogenesis. Because of the connections among all these flaws, PCOS is the outcome [6, 11]. We can prevent PCOS by losing weight because elevated BMI or fat deposition often speeds up insulin resistance and hyperandrogenism [11]. Hyperandrogenaemia is caused by an excess of androgen released by theca cells of the ovaries in response to the development of fat tissues [27]. Infertility, sadness, and anxiety are caused by the irregular menstrual cycle resulting from obesity and type 2 diabetes, which are caused by insulin resistance and hyperandrogen production [28].

Insulin resistance advances due to abnormal androgen synthesis caused by variations in the release of gonadotropin-releasing hormone (GnRH) release [24]. Follicle-stimulating hormone (FSH) is then lowered and luteinizing hormone (LH) is subsequently elevated when GnRH output is disrupted. Insulin enhances androgen synthesis in ovarian theca cells in conjunction with LH [24, 27]. Prior studies have demonstrated that insulin and LH work in concert to stimulate the synthesis and secretion of androgen by ovarian theca cells. However, because of some abnormalities in cortical steroidogenesis caused by an excess of adrenocorticotropic hormone (ACTH), the adrenal cortex produces an excessive amount of androgen [24, 28]. As an alternative, the cortex also produces testosterone. Hyperandrogenaemia stops the maturation of ovarian follicles and creates several small antral follicles [29]. This ultimately causes anovulation, which is characterised by elevated oestrogen levels resulting from the aromatase enzyme in peripheral adipose tissues converting androgen to oestrogen, while progesterone levels concurrently decline. One of the reasons for endometrial cancer is also the imbalance in sex hormones [27–30]. PCOS is a hormonal disorder characterised by abnormal ovarian and endometrial functions, primarily due to insulin resistance (IR), hyperandrogenism, excess oestrogen, and hyperinsulinemia [27, 29]. Factors such as genetics, environment, and obesity also contribute to the condition, affecting oocyte quality and endothelial function, leading to infertility and cardiovascular risks [31–33].

3.1 Hyperandrogen in polycystic ovary syndrome

Adrenocorticotropic hormone (ACTH) and luteinizing hormone (LH) are the primary sources of androgen in women [28]. The five forms of androgens include androstenedione (A4), testosterone (T), dihydrotestosterone (DHT), dehydroepiandrosterone (DHEA), and androstenedione sulphate (DHEAS) [31, 32]. The adrenal zona reticularis produces DHEAS, while the ovary and adrenal glands produce equal amounts of A4. DHEAS, DHEA, and A4 are precursors to testosterone. The liver metabolises all androgens, producing urine as the end product (**Figure 1**) [37, 38].

Ovarian theca cells biosynthesize testosterone from cholesterol, which is cleaved by enzymes P450 and CYP17A1 in the mitochondria [20, 26]. This leads to the conversion of pregnenolone into 17-hydroxypregnenolone, DHEA, and A4 [27, 31]. These substances are then converted into progesterone and 17-hydroxyprogesterone, respectively. 17β-hydroxysteroid dehydrogenase type 5 and CYP19A1 in granulosa cells convert A4 to testosterone and oestrone, while 5α-reductase and CYP19A1 convert testosterone to DHT and oestradiol (**Figure 2**) [32, 37].

DHT and testosterone are the two most active androgens available. DHT has three times the actions of testosterone [19]. Only 1% of testosterone is free, with the remaining 66% linked to sex hormone-binding globulin and 33% bound to albumin. It is interesting to note that protein-bound testosterone is inert, and only

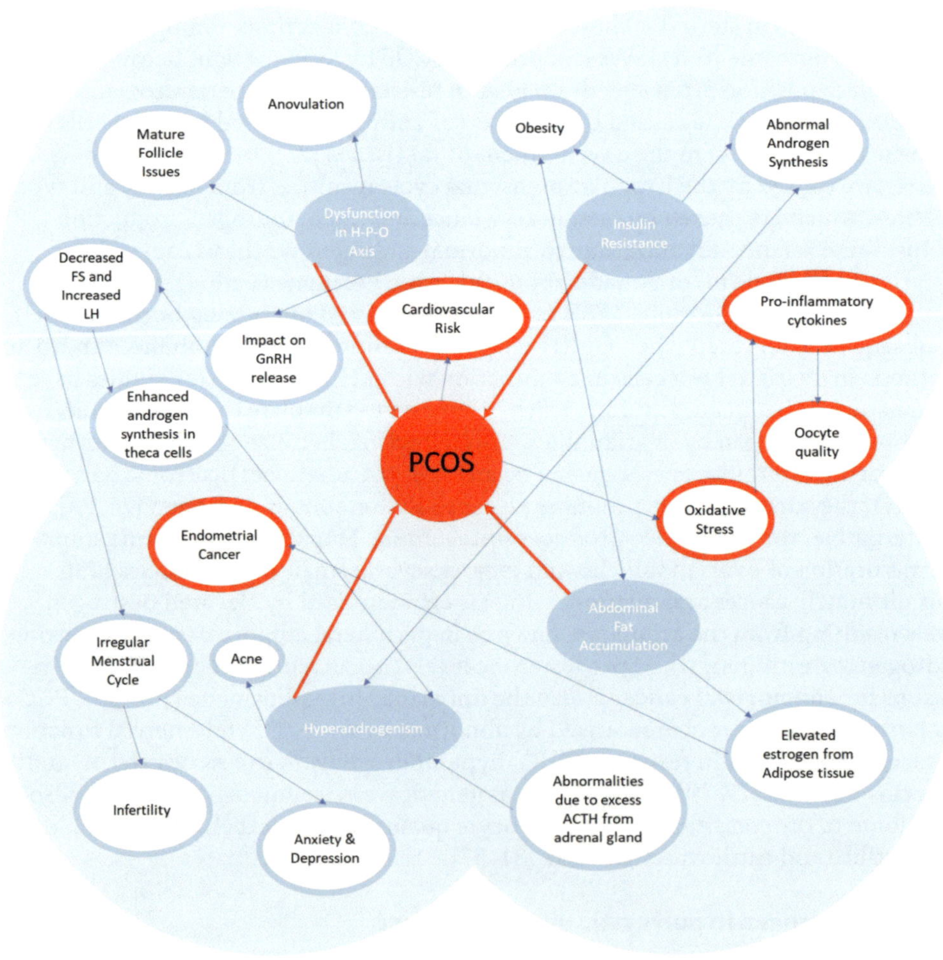

Figure 1.
Complex pathophysiology of PCOS [6, 11, 19–21, 24, 25, 27–47].

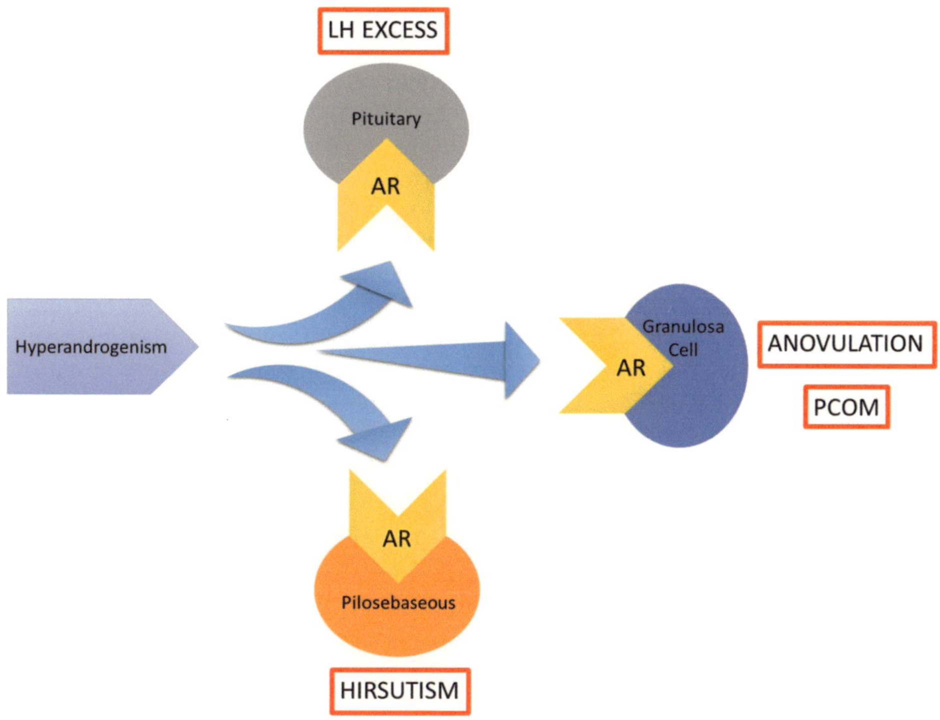

Figure 2.
Hyperandrogen and androgen receptor (AR) pathways [3, 11, 13, 17, 19–21, 24, 25, 27, 28, 31, 32, 34–43].

free testosterone exhibits biological activity. The only bioactive DHT is free DHT [19, 28]. Therefore, biological effects are caused by the levels of free testosterone and DHT in the blood. Androgen biological effects depend on their ability to bind to AR in tumour cells. Aromatase converts testosterone into oestrogen [38]. The female reproductive endocrine system is balanced by the cooperation of testosterone and oestradiol. Androgen contributes to increased muscle mass, bone growth, and calcium deposition in the peripheral organs [19, 38]. Adrenarche, or the release of androgens from the adrenal gland, is also necessary for developing pubic and axillary hair, which are signs of puberty. On the other hand, follicular dysplasia caused by high testosterone levels may hinder ovulation and cause menstrual problems [36]. Furthermore, androgens play a crucial role in maintaining a woman's sexual drive. Consequently, it is critical to preserve the equilibrium between androgen synthesis and secretion [38, 41].

The adrenal gland and ovaries are the primary sources of excess androgen, with 20–30% of PCOS patients experiencing adrenal hyperandrogenism [21]. The main cause of PCOS is an overabundance of androgens produced by the ovaries [24]. Four major GPCRs are associated with androgen production in PCOS patients' ovaries: the adrenocorticotropic hormone (ACTH)-specific melanocortin 2 receptor (MC2R), LH receptor (LHR), and FSH receptor (FSHR). The cAMP/PKA system is the primary signalling pathway regulating steroidogenesis [37, 42]. The AKT/PI3K pathway is a crucial non-gonadotropic signalling system linked to female reproductive disorders like PCOS [7, 21]. Overactivation of this pathway can lead to adipocyte differentiation, insulin resistance, and testosterone production [21, 37]. High expression levels of CYP17A1, CYP11A1, and StAR are associated with PCOS. Metformin, a treatment for PCOS-related complications, can attenuate androgen synthesis in theca cells by blocking PI3K/Akt signalling [32, 37].

Mitogen-activated protein kinase (MAPK) pathways are linked to various disorders, including PCOS. ERK1/2 is particularly linked to PCOS due to its role in androgen and oestrogen metabolism [28, 30]. The function of granulosa cells (GCs) affected by PCOS is reportedly affected by downregulation of phospho-ERK1/2 and MAPK kinase kinase 4 [31, 32]. Studies suggest that GCs' suppression of MAPK signalling causes CYP17 expression. The MAPK cascade may also suppress StAR and CYP17A1 expression. Further research is needed to understand the underlying mechanisms [32, 37, 42]. Wnt signalling, a process involved in cell growth, proliferation, migration, and death, has been found to play a significant role in polycystic ovary syndrome (PCOS) by stimulating androgen production [11, 17, 32]. Wnt4 mutations increase CYP11A1, CYP17, 17βHSD1, and StAR expression, affecting female sexuality and ovarian function. Further research is needed to determine Wnt4's contribution to PCOS and androgen hyperactivity. The signal pathways involved in androgen production create a complex network [36, 37, 42].

An additional crucial feature of PCOS patients is irregular menstrual cycles. The onset of the menstrual cycle is accompanied by an increase in anovulation, which can cause amenorrhoea, endometrial hyperproliferation, and even prostate cancer [3, 11]. When at least 12 antral follicles (AFC) with a diameter of 2–9 mm are distributed over the entire ovary and/or an ovarian volume greater than 10 mL, PCO is considered in women with PCOS [3, 13]. Overabundance of AFC may result in high levels of oestrogen secretion, which blocks the gonadal axis's negative feedback loop and prevents the release of follicle-stimulating hormone (FSH), causing anovulation [11, 28]. Thus, the two primary markers to assess the severity of PCOS are the length of the menstrual cycle and the quantity of ovaries' AFC [13]. The duration of the menstrual cycle and the number of AFC are positively correlated with serum testosterone levels, indicating that hyperandrogenism may contribute to the onset and progression of PCOS [3, 28]. Furthermore, excessive testosterone consumption can damage growth cones (GCs) and alter the follicle microenvironment, causing follicular atresia in PCOS [36].

Androgen plays a significant role in the development of oocytes in polycystic ovary syndrome (PCOS) [11, 17]. Overactive apoptosis, influenced by testosterone, can cause cell death through various signalling pathways [28]. This process is linked to abnormal microRNA production and the demethylation of programmed cell death [11, 27]. Additionally, androgen may directly cause oocyte death in PCOS [3, 17, 27]. Furthermore, androgens can inhibit the expression of growth and differentiation factor 9, preventing the transition from primary to secondary follicles and promoting primordial follicle activation [11, 36].

Autophagy plays a crucial role in folicle atresia, differentiation, and growth, and abnormal autophagy can affect oocyte growth and quality, leading to cell death [36, 38, 43]. In PCOS patients, excessive androgen intake can increase the ratio of autophagy markers and genes. Autophagy is disturbed in the ca cell layer, causing androgen synthesis and fibrosis through JNK/p38 and ROS signalling pathways [11, 17, 28]. Studies show that androgen excess can cause cell death, mitochondrial dysfunction, and the development of polycystic ovary syndrome (PCOS) [27, 28]. DHT may upregulate Drp1, a cytoplasmic GTPase involved in mitochondrial fission [36, 38]. This dysfunction affects energy metabolism and glycolytic metabolism, leading to low oocyte competence and dysfunctional GCs. Vitamin D3 can enhance mitochondrial dysfunction [38, 42, 43].

Endoplasmic reticulum stress, triggered by various physiological and pathological factors, affects cellular processes, including GCs [17, 24]. Excess testosterone can cause GCs to express UPR genes, leading to ER stress and cell apoptosis [30, 32]. Androgen-induced ER stress accumulates advanced glycation end products, intensifying PCOS's metabolic and reproductive effects. Resveratrol may be a therapeutic approach for PCOS patients and oocytes [33, 37].

High androgen levels during pregnancy may indicate PCOS, with prenatal androgenization (PNA) leading to endocrine characteristics like irregular oestrus cycles and resistance to progesterone [19, 20]. Premature births increase the risk of developing PCOS, visceral obesity, and early insulin resistance (IR) [25]. Anti-Müllerian hormone (AMH) levels are higher in newborns, children, and pre-puberty among women with PCOS [19, 30]. Obesity negatively impacts HA levels, but weight loss and lifestyle modifications can help women with PCOS maintain irregular reproductive patterns and metabolism. HA can also result in insulin resistance [25, 30, 32].

People with polycystic ovary syndrome (PCOS) have higher insulin receptor levels in their endometria, which can be influenced by long-term DHT therapy [32, 37]. Menstrual abnormalities, anovulation, and increased risk of endometrial hyperplasia and cancer are also common. Obesity may worsen these risk factors [37]. Overexpression of endometrial AR in PCOS patients triggers proinflammatory cytokines, and the onset of hyperplasia is linked to higher ERa and AR expression levels [20, 30, 37].

A4 is only partially released into the bloodstream, where it is converted in the skin and other peripheral tissues into androgens [38]. This can result in dermatological symptoms, such as acne, female pattern alopecia, and hirsutism, and excessive body or face hair [30]. The modified Ferriman-Gallwey (m-FG) score can be used to assess the severity of hirsutism [31]. In the vaginal skin of patients with PCOS, Stanczyk et al. more recently discovered an indirect DHT synthesis pathway [20, 21]. The first step in this process is the conversion of A4 to 5a-androstane-3,17-dione (5a-A) *via* 5a-reductase. HSD17B5 subsequently converts 5a-A into T [32]. The research has shown that despite, the fact that 5a-A and DHT are substantially lower in serum T and A4 concentrations, the vaginal tissue-to-serum ratios show the reverse effect [21, 31, 32]. Compared with the T and A4 groups, the 5a-A and DHT groups had substantially greater ratios. Therefore, the local conversion and metabolism of androgen are not entirely reflected in the androgen levels in circulation [21, 37, 38].

3.2 Insulin resistance in polycystic ovary syndrome

Metabolic alterations occur before reproductive abnormalities in PCOS, an autosomal dominant genetic illness with variable expression patterns that start in early childhood [24]. A clustering study of 893 women with PCOS identified the metabolic subtype of the disease, which was characterised by comparatively low SHBG and LH levels and increased BMI, glucose, and insulin levels [19]. One of the most notable phenotypic traits of PCOS is IR [29]. Twin and family cluster studies, revealed a hereditary component of PCOS related to HI, and substantial insulin secretion abnormalities were linked to a family history of T2DM [19, 29]. Before reaching puberty, the daughters of mothers with PCOS experience HI and decreased adiponectin levels, which last beyond adolescence [19, 24, 38].

PCOS is a condition characterised by specific gene mutations that regulate sheath steroid production, follicular maturation, and insulin signalling [24, 29]. Variants in the insulin receptor gene are strongly linked to insulin resistance (IR) in women with

PCOS [29, 38]. C/T polymorphisms in the INSR tyrosine kinase domain may contribute to compensatory hypoglycaemia and IR in normal-weight PCOS women [24, 38, 48]. The genetic makeup of insulin-related genes can also result from exposure to unfavourable intrauterine settings, such as dihydrotestosterone and insulin exposure during pregnancy [24, 29, 48].

Insulin is a hormone released by pancreatic beta cells that interacts with cell surface receptors [17, 23, 24, 29, 42]. Its α- and β-subunits form a heterotetramer, and its signal transduction is initiated by phosphorylation of intracellular substrates [24, 29, 34]. The two primary signalling routes for insulin are metabolism and mitosis [17, 42, 43]. The PI3-K pathway mediates metabolism, while the mitosis pathway involves the MAPK-ERK pathway [23, 24, 43, 48]. Insulin action can be stopped by increased serine phosphorylation and decreased tyrosine phosphorylation, leading to insulin failure in women with PCOS [34, 42, 44, 48].

Adipose tissue significantly influences insulin sensitivity and systemic glucose metabolism. Women with PCOS accumulate systemic fat and increase subcutaneous fat cell volume [34, 45, 48]. Whole-body insulin resistance (IR) is correlated with increased adipose tissue volume, with overconsumption of fatty acids causing lipid accumulation and intensifying insulin resistance [19, 25]. The study found that insulin-induced GLUT-4 in abdominal subcutaneous adipocytes with PCOS reduced, indicating defects in insulin receptor binding in adipocyte IR [25, 27, 28]. This suggests that androgens cause adipose tissue buildup and control lipid metabolism [24]. Exposure to androgens in animal models has been linked to increased adipocyte size, visceral fat deposition, and reduced insulin sensitivity in women [38]. High-molecular-weight adiponectin, a collagen-like protein, is adversely correlated with serum-free testosterone levels in PCOS [32, 34]. The dysfunction of adipose tissue may lead to low-level inflammation, insulin signal disruption, ectopic fat deposition, and insulin resistance [28, 42, 48].

Skeletal muscle, the most significant insulin-resistant tissue, is a key risk factor for type 2 diabetes in women with polycystic ovary syndrome (PCOS) [30]. Women with PCOS have lower insulin-mediated glucose digestion after meals, indicating poor insulin-stimulated glucose processing [31]. The molecular mechanisms underlying PCOS-specific insulin resistance in skeletal muscle are not yet established but include lipid buildup, signalling pathways, mitochondrial malfunction, genetic programming, and organ system interaction [41, 45]. Studies have shown that skeletal muscle insulin signalling deficiency may be PCOS-specific, and low circulating adiponectin levels may contribute to skeletal muscle insulin resistance [30, 46, 47].

Skeletal muscle biopsies of women with PCOS show that IR affects metabolic and mitotic pathways in the muscle [19]. Hyperandrogenaemia induces insulin resistance (IR) through fat storage and increased Akt/PKB, mTOR, and IRS1 serine phosphorylation [25, 39]. NF-κB activation can increase inflammation *via* hyperandrogenaemia [34]. Obesity is a predictor of skeletal muscle mass in women with PCOS, but not HA or IR [19, 39]. PCOS-specific IR is linked to abnormal gene expression and tissue crossing, with lower mitochondrial oxidative phosphorylation genes [19, 25, 34].

Postprandial glucose processing occurs in the liver, where insulin controls glucose uptake and storage [39]. Women with obesity often have PCOS-related hepatic insulin resistance, leading to impaired liver glycogen synthesis and glucose regulation [25]. Insulin growth factor 1 (IGF1) binding protein and liver SHBG production can be inhibited by IR and compensatory HI, causing hyperandrogenism and follicular development abnormalities [41]. Insulin action in fat and muscle indirectly affects glucose and lipid metabolism [48]. Insulin-mediated suppression of adipose tissue lipolysis raises circulating liver non-fatty acid levels, encouraging hepatic fat accumulation [19]. Insulin signalling is necessary for maintaining normal liver function and controlling glucose homoeostasis [20, 29]. Hepatic lipid accumulation intensifies hepatic insulin resistance (IR) by modulating insulin signalling and gluconeogenesis [19, 30]. Hepatic IR in female mice induced with hyperandrogenaemia is mediated by AR signalling in liver cells [34, 48]. Prolonged androgen excess can cause hepatic insulin resistance and steatosis, leading to non-alcoholic fatty liver disease (NAFLD). Liver IR is a significant risk factor for NAFLD in PCOS [20, 30, 48].

PCOS is primarily caused by ovarian androgen excess, with insulin-induced hysterectomy (HI) affecting follicular maturation and steroid production [35, 42, 43, 47]. Insulin signalling pathways regulate ovulation, and LH stimulates luteinization and boosts androgen production in membrane cells [24, 25, 43]. Androgen synthesis occurs in membrane cells, where insulin stimulates production by enhancing cytochrome P450c17α activity [9, 22, 47]. Women with PCOS are more vulnerable to hyperandrogenic effects of insulin, leading to premature LH receptor expression and granulosa cell differentiation [23, 24, 39]. Insulin resistance in ovarian tissue is linked to increased phosphorylation of MEk1/2 and MApK-ERk1/2 proteins [24, 35]. Endometrial function is affected by insulin resistance and hypoandrogenemia, with endometrial tissues lacking insulin receptors, IRS proteins, AS160, PKC, and GLUT4 [23, 35, 42]. Metformin, an insulin sensitizer, can help endometrial function in patients with PCOS by increasing AMPK and enhancing insulin resistance [22, 39, 47].

Insulin impacts the hypothalamic-pituitary system, raising GnRH gene expression, enhancing androgen biosynthesis, and decreasing ovarian function [32]. The central nervous system's insulin signalling is crucial for healthy reproduction and body weight control [37]. Insulin can directly increase LH production, leading to impaired reproductive function in PCOS patients [38, 47]. Disruption of pituitary insulin receptors and loss of pituitary sensitivity to GnRH can intensify hyperandrogenaemia and increase adrenal androgen levels [37, 47, 49]. Elevated leptin production by adipocytes contributes to insulin resistance (IR), and increased leptin expression in the hypothalamus can exacerbate obesity [32, 38, 47].

Epigenetic modifications, such as DNA methylation, histone status, and miRNA expression, control insulin resistance in women with polycystic ovary syndrome (PCOS) [11, 36, 46]. Hypermethylation of the LAMIN gene promoter is linked to insulin resistance [17, 39, 41]. MicroRNAs, crucial for androgen production, inflammation, and signalling, regulate gene expression [16, 39, 46]. MiRNA expression levels vary in women with PCOS and healthy women [36, 46]. Mir-155-5p and Mir-222 genes may be used as PCOS biomarkers [11, 16, 41]. Studies suggest that intestinal flora imbalance and bacteria metabolite levels can lead to insulin receptor signalling deficiency, causing insulin resistance (IR) by causing immune system dysfunction, chronic inflammation, and proinflammatory cytokine synthesis [11, 13, 29]. Vitamin D deficiency can intensify inflammatory responses and alter calcium homoeostasis, impacting insulin signalling [17, 29]. Melatonin regulation is linked to elevated insulin resistance, with MTNR1B signalling inhibiting insulin release in pancreatic beta cells. Prolonged stress can also promote visceral fat accumulation, resulting in insulin resistance [3, 11, 24].

The glucose clamp method is the gold standard for assessing metabolic insulin resistance *in vivo*. However, it is costly, labour-intensive, and not suitable for clinical settings [4, 12, 28]. Alternative quantitative indicators, such as anthropometric markers, oral glucose tolerance tests, and biomarkers, have been developed for clinical practice [29]. HOMA-IR is the most effective marker for diagnosing PCOS-IR, but more thorough assessments are needed [33]. Inflammatory indicators like ferritin and IL-6 are becoming more common in IR assessment, but their application in therapeutic contexts is limited by contradictory information [29, 44, 47].

3.3 Obesity and polycystic ovary syndrome

Polycystic ovary syndrome (PCOS) is linked to obesity, increasing the risk of developing type 2 diabetes, poor glucose tolerance, dyslipidaemia, and NAFLD [25, 47]. This cardiometabolic risk may lead to cardiovascular events and early death postmenopause [38]. However, there is limited data on PCOS-affected women postmenopause [42]. The primary cause of PCOS's hyperandrogenic and reproductive characteristics is the ovary's reaction to compensatory hyperinsulinemia, a malfunctioning PI3-K post-receptor insulin pathway influenced by body fat mass [29, 38, 47].

Adipose tissue releases adipokines, which are correlated with body fat amount and obesity [21, 31]. Visfatin, an adipokine involved in insulin sensitivity, inflammation, and metabolism, may contribute to metabolic dysfunction and insulin resistance in PCOS-affected women [32, 45]. However, research shows conflicting findings regarding various adipokines in PCOS, with retinol-binding protein 4 potentially modulating insulin sensitivity [32, 41, 45]. Future research should explore the mechanisms affecting serum adipokine impact on the PI3-K insulin pathway [31, 32, 41].

Hepatic and visceral fat levels are key mediators of insulin resistance and weight gain, particularly in women with polycystic ovary syndrome (PCOS) [2, 35, 41]. NAFLD is common in these women, suggesting hepatic fat may play a role [2, 25, 45]. However, recent research using MRI has challenged the notion that women with PCOS have more visceral fat [41, 48]. MRI-based research found equal visceral areas between groups, suggesting that visceral fat accumulation is a factor in PCOS insulin resistance and metabolic dysfunction [35, 41, 45].

Obesity, particularly abdominal phenotype, is a significant clinical predictor of metabolic syndrome in women with PCOS [16, 25, 36]. However, most studies are cross-sectional, retrospective, or case-control, limiting interpretation. Referral bias and cultural background can impact the prevalence of this condition [39, 41, 48]. Abdominal/visceral phenotype, excess body weight, and PCOS are prevalent in the PCOS community, exacerbated by lipid diseases, hypertension, glucose intolerance, and type 2 diabetes [14, 36, 39]. The altered function of visceral adipocytes in PCOS-affected women may lead to abnormal visceral fat formation [27, 41, 45]. Insulin resistance is negatively correlated with decreased high-molecular-weight adiponectin levels, which are linked to obesity and visceral fat expansion [27, 29, 32]. Low HMW-adiponectin levels are lower in PCOS, suggesting a harmful function for excess androgen [32, 41, 45]. Low-grade adipose tissue inflammation contributes to insulin resistance in PCOS, with visceral fat characterised by macrophage infiltration and inflammatory structures [27, 29, 45].

Insulin resistance in the arterial wall is linked to reduced nitric oxide synthesis, increased vascular stiffness, and impaired insulin vasodilatory action [7, 41]. This impairs insulin sensitivity in patients with PCOS and obesity [7]. Excessive insulin can cause hypertrophic vascular endothelium and smooth muscle cells, leading to endothelial dysfunction [29]. Insulin resistance, obesity, visceral fat, and type 2 diabetes are all linked to metabolic abnormalities, endothelial injury, vascular dysfunctions, and inflammation [27, 32, 36]. Studies show that dyslipidaemia is prevalent in PCOS-affected women, with supranormal non-HDL cholesterol levels, low HDL-C, and elevated triglyceride levels [6, 13]. These women have greater ApoCIII/ApoCII ratios and higher ApoCI levels. A clinical trial found that PCOS-affected women had a higher prevalence of metabolic syndrome, but low HDL-C levels were the only significant factor linked to PCOS [7, 20]. The normal profile of lipid disorder in PCOS remains controversial, largely influenced by visceral fatness and obesity [13, 25, 27]. Studies suggest that insulin resistance and obesity may influence altered lipid profiles in women with polycystic ovary syndrome (PCOS), particularly in the visceral phenotype [41]. Flutamide, a pure antiandrogen, can enhance lipid profiles, possibly due to the suppression of androgenic effects [15, 39]. Oxidative stress, defined by elevated free radical generation and reduced antioxidant levels, is also linked to PCOS [39, 41]. Advanced glycated end products (AGEs) play a significant role in PCOS, with elevated serum AGEs being a unique finding in women without obvious CV risk factors [15, 46, 48].

Studies on PCOS-related subclinical cardiovascular disease have shown that endothelial dysfunction is linked to increased testosterone levels and insulin resistance in women [5, 47, 50]. Women with PCOS have greater carotid intima-media thickness (CIMT) and higher rates of coronary artery calcification, suggesting a vascular insulin resistance state [5, 24]. Early atherosclerosis may result from lifetime exposure to an unfavourable CV risk profile in PCOS, with the link between CIMT and PCOS mainly explained by weight and fat distribution and related risk variables [23, 24, 50].

The relationship between PCOS and CVD events is unclear, and the current retrospective validation criteria for PCOS diagnoses are inconsistent [25]. Studies suggest a higher risk of CVD morbidity and mortality in women with irregular menstruation, but no current study shows a greater risk of myocardial infarction or stroke [47]. Further multicentre prospective studies are needed to assess the cardiovascular system in postmenopausal women with PCOS history [25, 39, 42].

4. Phenotypes of polycystic ovary syndrome

The National Institutes of Health (NIH) developed the diagnostic criteria for PCOS in 1990 [1]. These criteria included the presence of oligo/anovulation and clinical and/or biochemical hyperandrogenism [1, 7]. Three years ago, the ESHRE/ASRM Rotterdam Consensus included polycystic ovarian morphology (PCOM) on transvaginal ultrasonography as a third criterion [1, 2]. If all other potential explanations for the symptoms are ruled out, the patient must exhibit any two of the three characteristics listed in the Rotterdam criteria for PCOS to be diagnosed [2, 7]. Patients may be categorised into four main phenotypes based on the criteria met, each of which has a distinct clinical appearance: [1, 2, 16].

1. I—with oligo/anovulation, hyperandrogenism, and PCOM

2. II—with oligo/anovulation and hyperandrogenism

3. III—with hyperandrogenism and PCOM

4. IV—with oligo/anovulation and PCOM

The degree of metabolic problems varies among patients with PCOS and distinct phenotypes [2, 3]. Patients with normoandrogenic phenotypes are less likely to have metabolic problems than those with hyperandrogenism-associated phenotypes, regardless of ethnicity [7]. The metabolic profile of these individuals is exacerbated by intrinsic insulin resistance, which is strongly linked to NIH-defined PCOS characteristics [3, 7, 13]. Patients with a normoandrogenic phenotype have a milder metabolic profile than healthy women, but they also vary greatly from one another [3, 7]. PCOS metabolic abnormalities are mediated by inflammatory cytokines and adipokine and are linked to the combined effects of visceral obesity, insulin resistance, and hyperandrogenism [2, 13]. The variations observed across the four PCOS phenotypes highlight the necessity of an individualised approach to diagnosis and treatment [2, 3, 7].

5. Treatment of polycystic ovary syndrome

Crucially, no one-size-fits-all PCOS treatment is available; instead, care must always be customised to meet the unique needs of each patient [3, 51]. In mild cases requiring only proper follow-up of the patient's symptoms, treatment is symptom-oriented and may not be necessary at all (e.g., in a patient presenting with mild oligomenorrhea and PCOM) [7]. Actually, no medication has been licenced for the treatment of PCOS as of yet. Pharmacological therapy targets may include insulin resistance and androgen excess, but lifestyle counselling is the best course of action for preventing or treating obesity [3, 52]. A long-term, dynamic treatment plan that is tailored to each patient's unique needs, expectations, and changing circumstances is necessary for PCOS, as the disorder is lifelong, barring rare secondary cases in which the syndrome may resolve upon resolution of the triggering aetiological factor [3, 7, 51].

Anti-PCOS clinical therapy primarily addresses symptoms, but heavy pharmacological load increases the risk of metabolism-related issues [3, 51]. Oral contraceptives have serious side effects and are not long-term treatment choices [5]. Antiandrogen and androgen receptor modulators prevent androgens from acting, impairing libido and strength [3, 5]. GnRH antagonists are not recommended for PCOS patients undergoing infertility therapy, as they cause a shortage of oestrogen [52]. PCOS-related issues like insulin resistance, obesity, hirsutism, and acne are treated with unique medications [51–53].

International recommendations for treating PCOS include lifestyle adjustments to correct hyperinsulinemia, hormonal therapy, and combination oral contraceptives (COCs) [5, 51]. The World Health Organisation advises against using a combination of 35 μg of oestrogens and cyproterone acetate (CPA) for severe acne and hirsutism due to increased risk of thrombotic events [5, 14]. Women with metabolic syndrome or severe IR should not use contraceptives [13, 51]. Pharmaceuticals containing oestrogen-progestin contraceptive formulations help manage menstrual periods by increasing SHBG production and inhibiting androgen activity [3, 53]. Metformin is less effective than COCs and only slightly to moderately improves menstrual cycle regularity [10]. New recommendations call for a novel strategy promoting COCs in addition to metformin, particularly for overweight or obese women with PCOS [3, 12]. Current research shows no appreciable advantages of combining antiandrogenic medications with COCs [10, 53]. Future studies should focus on predicting accessibility and assessing the efficacy of combination medicines [3, 10].

PCOS diagnosis should be considered alongside comorbidities like obesity, type 2 diabetes, and mental distress [1, 53]. PCOS starts earlier than other women and increases the risk of these comorbidities [38]. Weight management is crucial, and new

DOI: http://dx.doi.org/10.5772/intechopen.1007169

guidelines recommend measuring waist circumference and checking weight regularly [51, 53]. Women with known risk factors for type 2 diabetes should undergo an oral glucose tolerance test every 1–3 years and have their HbA1c levels checked every 3 years [51]. Obesity is a high-risk factor for gestational diabetes in PCOS patients [1, 38, 53].

5.1 Lifestyle interventions

PCOS symptoms and weight control are suggested as the first line of treatment for obesity [12]. Weight-loss-oriented lifestyle treatments include dietary adjustments, physical activity, and behavioural therapies [13]. However, low-quality evidence supports these therapies, and they have only been tested in limited groups [38]. A 2019 study showed a 4-month intervention improved menstrual irregularity and weight loss but had no effect on ovulation or psychological health [54]. Patients with PCOS should follow a low-glycaemic index (GI) diet, focusing on controlling carbohydrate consumption and managing lipid profiles [5, 53]. Losing weight can improve menstrual cycle regulation, ovulation, cardiovascular system, and cancer risk [12, 33]. Maintaining fluid balance and balanced protein, fat, and carbohydrate meals is crucial [53, 54]. Excessive consumption of simple sugars has been linked to diabetes and cardiovascular issues [5, 53, 55]. High-fat ketogenic diets are not recommended for weight loss due to their restricted nature and potential mental health risks [5, 12, 55]. Short-term ketogenic diets combined with calorie restriction may be useful for treating PCOS, but further research is needed [12, 33].

Studies on exercise alone as a PCOS intervention have shown moderate evidence of lower BMI but no evidence of its influence on reproductive or hormonal outcomes [5, 8, 10]. Adherence to lifestyle changes is difficult, and adherence to trials is not significantly affected [8, 14]. A 47.1% attrition rate was found in four studies, but 63% experienced a weight drop of ≥5% [5, 19]. Behavioural support is recommended to address psychological issues associated with increased attrition [10, 14]. Overall, lifestyle interventions incorporating weight reduction have a good effect on PCOS metabolic characteristics, hyperandrogenism, and quality of life [14, 54, 55].

5.2 Medical interventions

The International PCOS guidelines recommend hirsutism, anovulation, and irregular cycles as treatment for the condition [4, 38]. Hyperandrogenism is a secondary treatment after lifestyle changes, and combination contraceptives (COCs) are recommended for treating hirsutism, acne, and irregular periods [5, 44, 51]. Metformin alone is less effective than COC treatment, but a combination of metformin and COCs is recommended, especially for overweight or obese women [4, 5, 44]. However, there is limited research on antiandrogen medication and the benefits of using a combination. Effective contraception is recommended for women with antiandrogens [44, 51].

Letrozole is recommended as the first-line therapy for women with PCOS and infertility, as it enhances live birth and clinical pregnancy rates and shortens the time to conception compared to clomiphene citrate [6, 7, 51]. However, metformin has a negligible positive effect on ovulation and live birth compared to placebo [3, 4]. Future research should focus on metformin priming before letrozole ovulation induction [6, 14, 51].

Metformin is used to improve hormonal, metabolic, and reproductive functions in individuals with PCOS and IR, while decreasing liver glucose production and increasing insulin sensitivity [13, 42, 51]. However, it may cause side effects and be contraindicated for severe conditions [5, 6, 12].

Antiandrogen therapy is a safer solution for women with IR or metabolic syndrome, reducing excess androgen levels and causing symptoms of high androgen levels [5, 39]. Two categories of antiandrogens are 5-alpha reductase inhibitors like finasteride and androgen receptor antagonists like spironolactone and flutamide [6, 8]. Combination with metformin may help manage obesity and enhance glucose tolerance [12, 13]. Spironolactone is used for acne and hirsutism but has side effects like gynaecomastia [5, 6, 38]. Propecia® is another antiandrogen used for acne and hirsutism but has side effects like reduced libido and erectile dysfunction [6, 8, 13]. Pregnancy and intolerance to the product are contraindications [12, 38, 39].

5.3 Surgical interventions

Sometimes, PCOS-related symptoms can be relieved by surgery [3]. When all other treatment options have failed, bariatric surgery is an excellent treatment option for obesity and PCOS, and patients who are extremely obese should be offered this option [5, 6]. However, surgery and diet are associated with risks, and pregnancy should not be attempted for a full year after the procedure [10, 12]. To restore and enhance ovarian function in patients with PCOS, laparoscopic ovarian drilling is a minimally invasive laparoscopic method that involves destroying ovarian tissue with a laser beam or surgical needle [15]. This process is not widely employed, but it is still a possibility in situations where the ovaries are resistant to clomiphene citrate and in situations where letrozole is not an option because of off-label use [5, 10, 15]. However, according to a recent Cochrane Review, compared with medical ovulation induction alone, laparoscopic ovarian drilling may actually lower the live birth rate in women with anovulatory PCOS and clomiphene citrate resistance, while also lowering the number of multiple pregnancies and the risk of ovarian hyperstimulation syndrome [3, 10, 38, 51].

6. Conclusions

The underlying aetiology of PCOS remains unclear despite the use of a number of treatment strategies to address the condition and its consequences. As a result, the opportunity for further research is in comprehensive mechanistic studies to identify the cause of and treat PCOS. The primary goal of current treatment is to relieve patients of the symptoms caused by different consequences related to hyperandrogenism. Consequently, decreasing the drug load of medications that patients are taking individually for various symptoms related to numerous problems may be made easier by utilising therapeutic targets such as 17b-HSD5, PTP1B, and NK3Rs to treat the underlying cause of difficulties. PTP1B contributes to the development of obesity and insulin resistance in diabetes mellitus.

Consequently, PTP1B inhibitor therapy may help control obesity and diabetes, thereby lowering the need for individual medication for each pathological disease. In addition to medication, attempts to assist patients with PCOS in changing their lifestyle choices will help lower the disease's risk and pace of development. There are established strategies to lessen the severity of the illness, such as eating a balanced diet, exercising, and getting enough sleep. The use of plant-produced items and their impact on PCOS are the subjects of much investigation. However, further research is needed to identify the ingredients that lead to these plants' positive benefits, which will hasten the proper application of these commodities.

Acknowledgements

The authors would like to extend a special thanks to Prof. Dr. M. Ahmad Djojosugito, SpOT (K) MHA, for providing support.

The study received no extramural funding.

Conflict of interest

The authors declare no conflict of interest.

Author details

I Gusti Agung Ngurah Agung Sentosa[1*] and Angel Benny Wisan[2]

1 Department of Obstetrics and Gynaecology, Faculty of Medicine, Ganesha University of Education, Singaraja, Bali, Indonesia

2 Department of Dermatology and Venereology, Faculty of Medicine, Mahasaraswati University, Denpasar, Bali, Indonesia

*Address all correspondence to: ign.agung.sentosa@undiksha.ac.id

References

[1] Escobar-Morreale HF. Polycystic ovary syndrome: Definition, aetiology, diagnosis and treatment. Nature Reviews Endocrinology. 2018;**14**(5):270-284. DOI: 10.1038/nrendo.2018.24

[2] Belenkaia LV, Lazareva LM, Walker W, Lizneva DV, Suturina LV. Criteria, phenotypes and prevalence of polycystic ovary syndrome. Minerva Ginecologica. 2019;**71**(3):211-225. DOI: 10.23736/S0026-4784.19.04404-6

[3] Hoeger KM, Dokras A, Piltonen T. Update on PCOS: Consequences, challenges, and guiding treatment. The Journal of Clinical Endocrinology and Metabolism. 2021;**106**(3):E1071-E1083. DOI: 10.1210/clinem/dgaa839

[4] Islam H, Masud J, Islam YN, Haque FKM. An update on polycystic ovary syndrome: A review of the current state of knowledge in diagnosis, genetic etiology, and emerging treatment options. Women's Health (London, England). 2022;**18**:1-23. DOI: 10.1177/17455057221117966

[5] Mimouni NEH, Giacobini P. Polycystic ovary syndrome (PCOS): Progress towards a better understanding and treatment of the syndrome. Comptes Rendus Biologies. 2024;**347**(G1):19-25. DOI: 10.5802/crbiol.147

[6] Kulkarni S et al. Polycystic ovary syndrome: Current scenario and future insights. Drug Discovery Today. 2023;**28**(12):1-15. DOI: 10.1016/j.drudis.2023.103821

[7] Aversa A et al. Fundamental concepts and novel aspects of polycystic ovarian syndrome: Expert consensus resolutions. Frontiers in Endocrinology (Lausanne). 2020;**11**:1-16. DOI: 10.3389/fendo.2020.00516

[8] Witchel SF, Burghard AC, Tao RH, Oberfield SE. The diagnosis and treatment of PCOS in adolescents: An update. Current Opinion in Pediatrics. 2019;**31**(4):562-569. DOI: 10.1097/MOP.0000000000000778

[9] Dabadghao P. Polycystic ovary syndrome in adolescents. Best Practice & Research. Clinical Endocrinology & Metabolism. 2019;**33**(3):101272. DOI: 10.1016/j.beem.2019.04.006

[10] Kostopoulou E, Anagnostis P, Bosdou JK, Spiliotis BE, Goulis DG. Polycystic ovary syndrome in adolescents: Pitfalls in diagnosis and management. Current Obesity Reports. 2020;**9**(3):193-203. DOI: 10.1007/s13679-020-00388-9

[11] Siddiqui S, Mateen S, Ahmad R, Moin S. A brief insight into the etiology, genetics, and immunology of polycystic ovarian syndrome (PCOS). Journal of Assisted Reproduction and Genetics. 2022;**39**(11):2439-2473. DOI: 10.1007/s10815-022-02625-7

[12] Stańczak NA, Grywalska E, Dudzińska E. The latest reports and treatment methods on polycystic ovary syndrome. Annals of Medicine. 2024;**56**(1):1-21. DOI: 10.1080/07853890.2024.2357737

[13] Collée J, Mawet M, Tebache L, Nisolle M, Brichant G. Polycystic ovarian syndrome and infertility: Overview and insights of the putative treatments. Gynecological Endocrinology. 2021;**37**(10):869-874. DOI: 10.1080/09513590.2021.1958310

[14] Glueck CJ, Goldenberg N. Characteristics of obesity in polycystic ovary syndrome: Etiology, treatment,

and genetics. Metabolism. 2019;**92**:108-120. DOI: 10.1016/j.metabol.2018.11.002

[15] Ganie MA, Vasudevan V, Wani IA, Baba MS, Arif T, Rashid A. Epidemiology, pathogenesis, genetics & management of polycystic ovary syndrome in India. The Indian Journal of Medical Research. 2019;**150**(4):333-344. DOI: 10.4103/ijmr.IJMR_1937_17

[16] Kim JJ, Choi YM. Phenotype and genotype of polycystic ovary syndrome in Asia: Ethnic differences. The Journal of Obstetrics and Gynaecology Research. 2019;**45**(12):2330-2337. DOI: 10.1111/jog.14132

[17] Combs JC, Hill MJ, Decherney AH. Polycystic ovarian syndrome genetics and epigenetics. Clinical Obstetrics and Gynecology. 2021;**64**(1):20-25. DOI: 10.1097/GRF.0000000000000581

[18] Mumusoglu S, Yildiz BO. Polycystic ovary syndrome phenotypes and prevalence: Differential impact of diagnostic criteria and clinical versus unselected population. Current Opinion in Endocrine and Metabolic Research. 2020;**12**:66-71. DOI: 10.1016/j.coemr.2020.03.004

[19] Wang J, Wu D, Guo H, Li M. Hyperandrogenemia and insulin resistance: The chief culprit of polycystic ovary syndrome. Life Sciences. 2019;**236**:1-9. DOI: 10.1016/j.lfs.2019.116940

[20] Abbott DH, Dumesic DA, Levine JE. Hyperandrogenic origins of polycystic ovary syndrome – Implications for pathophysiology and therapy. Expert Review of Endocrinology and Metabolism. 2019;**14**(2):131-143. DOI: 10.1080/17446651.2019.1576522

[21] Ye W, Xie T, Song Y, Zhou L. The role of androgen and its related signals in PCOS. Journal of Cellular and Molecular Medicine. 2021;**25**(4):1825-1837. DOI: 10.1111/jcmm.16205

[22] Dumont A, Robin G, Dewailly D. Anti-müllerian hormone in the pathophysiology and diagnosis of polycystic ovarian syndrome. Current Opinion in Endocrinology, Diabetes, and Obesity. 2018;**25**(6):377-384. DOI: 10.1097/MED.0000000000000445

[23] Sahmay S, Aydogan Mathyk B, Sofiyeva N, Atakul N, Azemi A, Erel T. Serum AMH levels and insulin resistance in women with PCOS. European Journal of Obstetrics, Gynecology, and Reproductive Biology. 2018;**224**:159-164. DOI: 10.1016/j.ejogrb.2018.03.007

[24] Zhao H, Zhang J, Cheng X, Nie X, He B. Insulin resistance in polycystic ovary syndrome across various tissues: An updated review of pathogenesis, evaluation, and treatment. Journal of Ovarian Research. 2023;**16**(1):1-17. DOI: 10.1186/s13048-022-01091-0

[25] Pasquali R. Metabolic syndrome in polycystic ovary syndrome. Frontiers of Hormone Research. 2018;**49**:114-130. DOI: 10.1159/000485995

[26] Walters KA. Polycystic ovary syndrome: Is it androgen or estrogen receptor? Current Opinion in Endocrine and Metabolic Research. 2020;**12**:1-7. DOI: 10.1016/j.coemr.2020.01.003

[27] Fahs D, Salloum D, Nasrallah M, Ghazeeri G. Polycystic ovary syndrome: Pathophysiology and controversies in diagnosis. Diagnostics. 2023;**13**(9):1-13. DOI: 10.3390/diagnostics13091559

[28] Tsai YR, Liao YN, Kang HY. Current advances in cellular approaches for pathophysiology and treatment of polycystic ovary syndrome. Cells.

2023;**12**(17):1-26. DOI: 10.3390/cells12172189

[29] Herman R, Sikonja J, Jensterle M, Janez A, Dolzan V. Insulin metabolism in polycystic ovary syndrome: Secretion, signaling, and clearance. International Journal of Molecular Sciences. 2023;**24**(4):3140. DOI: 10.3390/ijms24043140

[30] Xu Y, Qiao J. Association of insulin resistance and elevated androgen levels with polycystic ovarian syndrome (PCOS): A review of literature. Journal of Healthcare Engineering. 2022;**2022**: 1-13. DOI: 10.1155/2022/9240569

[31] De Medeiros SF, Rodgers RJ, Norman RJ. Adipocyte and steroidogenic cell cross-talk in polycystic ovary syndrome. Human Reproduction Update. 2021;**27**(4):771-796. DOI: 10.1093/humupd/dmab004

[32] Zeng X, Xie YJ, Liu YT, Long SL, Mo ZC. Polycystic ovarian syndrome: Correlation between hyperandrogenism, insulin resistance and obesity. Clinica Chimica Acta. 2020;**502**:214-221. DOI: 10.1016/j.cca.2019.11.003

[33] Bhattacharya K et al. Polycystic ovary syndrome and its management: In view of oxidative stress. Biomolecular Concepts. 2024;**15**(1):1-21. DOI: 10.1515/bmc-2022-0038

[34] Li Y et al. Multi-system reproductive metabolic disorder: Significance for the pathogenesis and therapy of polycystic ovary syndrome (PCOS). Life Sciences. 2019;**228**:167-175. DOI: 10.1016/j.lfs.2019.04.046

[35] Walters KA, Gilchrist RB, Ledger WL, Teede HJ, Handelsman DJ, Campbell RE. New perspectives on the pathogenesis of PCOS: Neuroendocrine origins. Trends in Endocrinology and Metabolism. 2018;**29**:841-852. DOI: 10.1016/j.tem.2018.08.005

[36] Macut D, Bjekić-Macut J, Rahelić D, Doknić M. Insulin and the polycystic ovary syndrome. Diabetes Research and Clinical Practice. 2017;**130**:163-170. DOI: 10.1016/j.diabres.2017.06.011

[37] Wang K, Li Y, Chen Y. Androgen excess: A hallmark of polycystic ovary syndrome. Frontiers in Endocrinology (Lausanne). 2023;**14**:1-15. DOI: 10.3389/fendo.2023.1273542

[38] Armanini D, Boscaro M, Bordin L, Sabbadin C. Controversies in the pathogenesis, diagnosis and treatment of PCOS: Focus on insulin resistance, inflammation, and Hyperandrogenism. International Journal of Molecular Sciences. 2022;**23**(8):1-12. DOI: 10.3390/ijms23084110

[39] Rudnicka E et al. Anti-müllerian hormone in pathogenesis, diagnostic and treatment of PCOS. International Journal of Molecular Sciences. 2021;**22**(22):1-12. DOI: 10.3390/ijms222212507

[40] Rosenfield RL. Current concepts of polycystic ovary syndrome pathogenesis. Current Opinion in Pediatrics. 2020;**32**(5):698-706. DOI: 10.1097/MOP.0000000000000945

[41] Barber TM, Franks S. Obesity and polycystic ovary syndrome. Clinical Endocrinology. 2021;**95**(4):531-541. DOI: 10.1111/cen.14421

[42] Wang K, Li Y. Signaling pathways and targeted therapeutic strategies for polycystic ovary syndrome. Frontiers in Endocrinology (Lausanne). 2023;**14**:1-28. DOI: 10.3389/fendo.2023.1191759

[43] Zhang J, Bao Y, Zhou X, Zheng L. Polycystic ovary syndrome and mitochondrial dysfunction. Reproductive

Biology and Endocrinology. 2019;**17**(1): 1-15. DOI: 10.1186/s12958-019-0509-4

[44] Notaro ALG, Neto FTL. The use of metformin in women with polycystic ovary syndrome: An updated review. Journal of Assisted Reproduction and Genetics. 2022;**39**(3):573-579. DOI: 10.1007/s10815-022-02429-9

[45] Dumesic DA, Abbott DH, Sanchita S, Chazenbalk GD. Endocrine–metabolic dysfunction in polycystic ovary syndrome: An evolutionary perspective. Current Opinion in Endocrine and Metabolic Research. 2020;**12**:41-48. DOI: 10.1016/j.coemr.2020.02.013

[46] Yurtdaş G, Akdevelioğlu Y. A new approach to polycystic ovary syndrome: The gut microbiota. Journal of the American College of Nutrition. 2020;**39**(4):371-382. DOI: 10.1080/07315724.2019.1657515

[47] Krentowska A, Kowalska I. Metabolic syndrome and its components in different phenotypes of polycystic ovary syndrome. Diabetes/Metabolism Research and Reviews. 2022;**38**(1):e3464. DOI: 10.1002/dmrr.3464

[48] He FF, Li YM. Role of gut microbiota in the development of insulin resistance and the mechanism underlying polycystic ovary syndrome: A review. Journal of Ovarian Research. 2020;**13**(1):1-13. DOI: 10.1186/s13048-020-00670-3

[49] McCartney CR, Campbell RE. Abnormal GnRH pulsatility in polycystic ovary syndrome: Recent insights. Current Opinion in Endocrine and Metabolic Research. 2020;**12**:78-84. DOI: 10.1016/j.coemr.2020.04.005

[50] Dabravolski SA et al. Mitochondrial dysfunction and chronic inflammation in polycystic ovary syndrome. International Journal of Molecular Sciences. 2021;**22**(8):1-20. DOI: 10.3390/ijms22083923

[51] Jin P, Xie Y. Treatment strategies for women with polycystic ovary syndrome. Gynecological Endocrinology. 2018;**34**(4):272-277. DOI: 10.1080/09513590.2017.1395841

[52] Della Corte L et al. Current and experimental drug therapy for the treatment of polycystic ovarian syndrome. Expert Opinion on Investigational Drugs. 2020;**29**(8):819-830. DOI: 10.1080/13543784.2020.1781815

[53] Glintborg D, Andersen M. Medical treatment and comorbidity in polycystic ovary syndrome: An updated review. Current Opinion in Endocrine and Metabolic Research. 2020;**12**:33-40. DOI: 10.1016/j.coemr.2020.02.014

[54] Colombo GE, Pirotta S, Sabag A. Diet and exercise in the Management of Polycystic Ovary Syndrome: Practical considerations for person-Centered care. Seminars in Reproductive Medicine. 2023;**41**(1-2):26-36. DOI: 10.1055/s-0043-1777116

[55] Han Y et al. Effect of high fat diet on disease development of polycystic ovary syndrome and lifestyle intervention strategies. Nutrients. 2023;**15**(9):1-14. DOI: 10.3390/nu15092230

Section 4

Estrogens

Chapter 6

Reproductive Landmarks and Lipedema: Lessons to be Learned about Women Hormones throughout Life

Juliana Bicca

Abstract

Lipedema is an old disease that just recently is being reconized and causes huge interest. Because it eminently affects women, its pathophysiology has always been related to estradiol. Understanding the mechanisms that start the disease and make it progress throughout life points toward that it is a disease related to women's reproductive milestones: menarch, pregnancy and menopause. But what is common in women's reproductive milestones that places them at a greater risk of developing Lipedema? Menarch, pregnancy and menopause are phases of a woman's life that have little similarity from the hormonal point of view: where in one, the estrogens are high, and in the other, they are low; where in one, the FSH/LH is low, and in another, those levels may be strictly high. The proposal of this chapter also includes the impact of hormonal metabolomics in adipose tissue and adipocyte intracrinology to women's health throughout her reproductive life.

Keywords: Lipedema, reproductive landmarks, hormones, estradiol, inflammation

1. Introduction

Hormonal changes play a crucial role in the development and progression of Lipedema, a chronic condition that mainly affects women.

Understanding how female hormones affect adipose tissue and the distribution of fat in the body is fundamental to the proper management of this disease. In addition, the production of sex steroids in both normal and abnormal adipose tissue may influence the pathophysiology of Lipedema and potentially open up new treatment alternatives.

Normal adipose tissue is both hormone-active (hormone-producing) and hormone-sensitive (hormone-responsive) in Lipedema, a complex, hormonal and inflammatory disease of adipose and connective tissue. It becomes even more important that we can better understand the impact of hormonal dysfunctions throughout a woman's reproductive life—with or without Lipedema. Lipedema therefore becomes a biological model for us to gain a deeper understanding of sex steroid hormones and their impact throughout a woman's reproductive life.

Throughout a woman's life, from puberty to menopause, the hormonal changes that occur during reproductive milestones have a significant impact on Lipedema. Understanding these hormonal changes and their effect on adipose tissue provides valuable insights into the clinical and therapeutic approach to this very prevalent condition. Lipedema has mistakenly been described as a disease that arises or progresses in association with hormonal peaks. This does not seem to be true, and so this author suggests that we come to understand Lipedema as a disease associated with female reproductive milestones so that we can also understand the marked differences between these moments.

It is important to consider not only the traditional sex hormones, such as estrogen and progesterone, but also other hormonal mediators, such as thyroid hormones, insulin, cortisol and GH, which also play a role in metabolism, body weight regulation and the distribution of body fat in humans.

Up to 60% of women with Lipedema are also obese, and the effect of obesity on female fertility has long been well recognized. In addition, a recent study found that women with lipedema can present with unusual higher infertility rates.

An in-depth study of hormonal changes in the reproductive milestones of women with Lipedema is essential if we are to advance our knowledge of this complex disease and develop more effective and personalized treatment strategies. The interaction between female hormones and the abnormal adipose tissue of Lipedema opens up new research and therapeutic perspectives, with the potential to improve the quality of life of women affected by Lipedema.

2. Reproductive milestones

According to the Stages of Reproductive Aging Workshop (STRAW), a woman's reproductive life is defined in seven stages ranging from menarche to the menopausal transition and post-menopausal phases.

A woman's reproductive milestones play a crucial role in the changes in the biological behavior of adipose tissue in Lipedema. During different phases of a woman's reproductive life, such as puberty, pregnancy and menopause, significant hormonal changes occur, guided by variations in FSH and LH and their impact on the regulation of both gonadal and extra-gonadal steroidogenesis, which influence the distribution of fat in the body and can play a role in the development and progression of Lipedema.

Although men and women show differences in body composition from birth, it is the onset of puberty and the influence of sex hormones that ultimately determine the distribution of body fat in women. But animal models show us that not only the quantities or cyclicity with which they are produced but also the biological responses of adipose tissue to sex steroids, which are also determined by the distribution and type of estrogen receptors (ER alpha and beta), expression of steroidogenesis enzymes (e.g., aromatase) and the presence of FSH-responsive elements [1].

The distribution of body fat in women, among other factors, is intensely influenced by estrogens, which is why their importance in the pathophysiology of Lipedema is emphasized (effect of ovariectomy on adipose tissue of mice in the absence of estrogen receptor alpha: a potential role for estrogen receptor beta).

Puberty is a phase marked by the beginning of reproductive cycles with cyclical elevations of gonadotropins that will lead to the two phases of the female menstrual cycle—the first is characterized by the progressive elevation of estradiol while the second by ovulation and elevation of progesterone. These hormonal changes not only determine a woman's reproductive capacity but also determine the distribution of fat in the female body, particularly in subcutaneous adipose tissue with a gynoid predominance, such as the gluteus femoris region—the areas most classically affected by Lipedema. Most women with Lipedema report an onset of symptoms during or after puberty, suggesting that this phase is an important milestone in the history of the disease. With the onset of menstrual cycles, there are monthly fluctuations in FSH and LH levels, related to cyclical fluctuations in estradiol and progesterone.

During pregnancy, hormonal changes are even more pronounced, with a significant increase in estrogen and progesterone levels to support pregnancy at levels that a woman would never normally experience at other stages of her life. In parallel, pituitary FSH and LH are suppressed as pituitary production of gonadotropins is replaced by placental control under the effect of human chorionic gonadotropin. During pregnancy, the preferential storage pattern of gluteofemoral fat becomes amplified, with increased fat storage and lipolysis resistance [2].

In addition, during pregnancy, we have the additional effect of an insulin resistance status, especially from the second trimester onward, which favors fat deposition and inhibits lipolysis.

Interestingly, gluteal-femoral fat cells are practically unresponsive to catecholamines in pregnancy [3].

Lassek and Gaulin [4] demonstrated that gluteofemoral fat is important for infant neural development, reporting that gluteofemoral fat accounts for 60 to 80% of the amount of long-chain polyunsaturated fatty acids (LCFA), especially omega-3 (dha), in breast milk.

During pregnancy and lactation, prolactin, a hormone produced by lactotrophs in the anterior pituitary gland, also comes into play. There are reports of Lipedema associated with pituitary tumors and some cases of Lipedema associated with PIT1 mutation and GH deficiency, which could probably be associated with a Lipedema phenotype linked to pituitary dysfunction. PRL receptors have also been characterized in adipose tissue, regulating adipogenesis and inhibiting lipolysis. During lactation and pregnancy, there is an increase in the expression of prolactin receptors, which may at least partly explain the progression of Lipedema during these phases [5].

During pregnancy, once again, hormones will determine a very characteristic distribution of body fat with an even more pronounced accumulation of adipose tissue in the gluteal-femoral regions in order to keep energy reserves safe for the maintenance of maternal-fetal health.

Studies also suggest that Lipedema can manifest for the first time or worsen during pregnancy, highlighting the influence of reproductive hormones in this context.

Finally, during the menopausal transition and menopause, which mark the end of a woman's reproductive life, there is a progressive decrease in the production of estrogen and progesterone and an increase in FSH and LH levels. This hormonal transition again impacts body fat distribution and the function of adipose tissue, which undergoes changes in order to take over steroidogenesis once this function performed by the ovaries progressively declines until it ceases, potentially impacting the progression of Lipedema. About 67% of women who enter menopause with Lipedema report a worsening of the condition, which highlights the importance of better understanding the impact of extra-gonadal steroidogenesis on the pathophysiology and progression of the disease at this reproductive milestone.

It should be noted, therefore, how different the phases of a woman's life are from the hormonal point of view, where the peaks of worsening Lipedema are

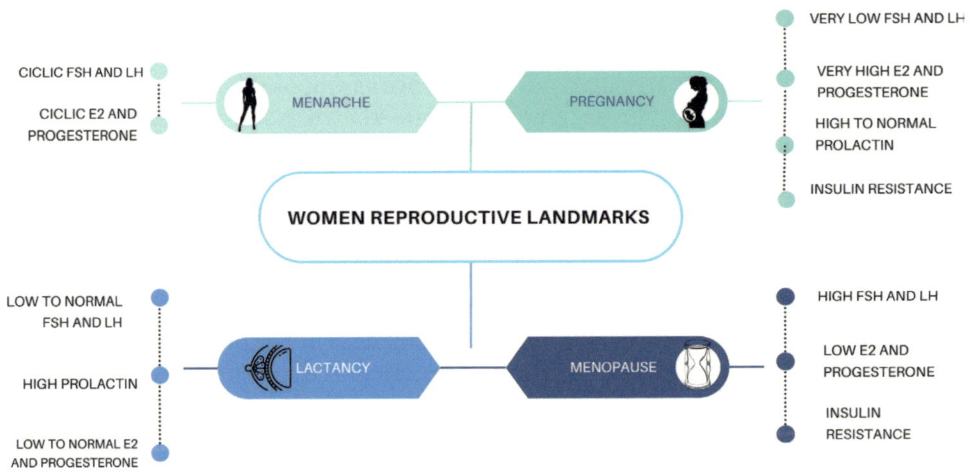

Figure 1.
Reproductive landmarks and hormonal changes related to Lipedema.

classically observed, and that it is the hormones—FSH, LH, prolactin, HCG, androgens and not just estrogens—that are the major triggers for the evolution and progression of the disease, allowing us to define Lipedema in many ways as a hormonal and inflammatory disease of adipose tissue. In women, it is hormones and not genetics that determine how our bodies modify their fat distribution throughout life (**Figure 1**).

One thing that needs to be analyzed alongside hormonal changes is the influence of the inflammation found in this diseased adipose tissue since it can be very difficult to understand whether it is the inflamed adipose tissue that generates more local estrogen or whether it is the local estrogenic changes that generate more inflammation? In fact, the relationship between estrogen and inflammation is extremely complex and depends on the type of inflammation stimulus, cell type, reproductive status (pre-menopause, post-menopause, pregnancy), total estrogen load (total, serum and tissue estrogen concentration), estrogen receptor expression, local estrogen metabolism, estrogen effects on the hypothalamic-pituitary-adrenal axis, estrogen effect on the peripheral nervous system and sympathetic activation [6].

Understanding Lipedema requires a broad and in-depth view of the hormonal behavior of adipose tissue as a major endocrine organ.

3. Steroidogenesis in adipose tissue and intracrinology

Steroidogenesis in women's adipose tissue is a complex and fundamental process for the regulation of sex steroids, such as the female sex hormones (estrogen and progesterone) and their precursors, in the female organism. Adipose tissue is not only an energy storage site but also an important endocrine gland capable of producing and metabolizing steroid hormones.

The evolution of hormonal systems over 500 million years has allowed the expression of more than 30 steroid hormone-forming enzymes to be expressed in non-gonadal peripheral tissues, allowing steroid synthesis to be maintained at the cellular level. In women, the main representative of extra-gonadal steroidogenesis is adipose tissue.

The ability of adipose tissue to convert steroid precursors, such as cholesterol, into sex hormones occurs through a series of enzymatic reactions known as steroidogenesis. The enzymes involved in this process are expressed in adipose tissue, enabling the local biosynthesis of steroid hormones. This means that fat cells have the ability to produce sex steroids from precursor molecules, contributing to female hormone regulation.

Intracrinology, a concept closely related to steroidogenesis in adipose tissue, refers to the production, metabolism and action of hormones at a tissue level, without the need for systemic production in the ovaries or adrenal glands. In the female context, intracrinology plays a crucial role in regulating the levels and action of sex hormones, especially during phases of reproductive life such as menopause.

The importance of this phenomenon in female hormonal health is significant. The ability of adipose tissue to produce sex steroids locally directly impacts various physiological processes, such as the menstrual cycle, fertility, body composition and women's metabolic health. Imbalances in steroidogenesis in adipose tissue can result in altered levels of sex hormones, leading to hormonal disorders such as polycystic ovary syndrome and menopausal complications.

In addition, intracrinology in adipose tissue plays an important role in the development and progression of metabolic and endocrine disorders, such as insulin resistance, obesity and even the progression of certain hormone-related cancers, such as breast cancer. Therefore, understanding and considering steroidogenesis in adipose tissue and intracrinology when assessing female hormonal health is essential for comprehensive and effective care.

In lipedemic adipocytes, alterations in the expression and activity of local steroidogenesis enzymes may have significant implications. Evidence suggests that chronic inflammation, often present in Lipedema, can negatively impact the regulation of estrogen metabolism. Inflammatory cytokines such as TNF-α and IL-6 are known to suppress aromatase expression, resulting in lower local estrogen production. This effect can contribute to a hormonal imbalance, exacerbating the abnormal fat accumulation and metabolic dysfunction seen in Lipedema. Estrogen, particularly estradiol, plays an important role in the metabolic regulation and distribution of adipose tissue in women and the loss of this protective mechanism may be involved in Lipedema. In addition, it is possible that locally there are also changes in estrogen metabolism that favor the generation of estrogen metabolites that negatively influence adipogenesis, such as 16-oh estrone and 4-oh estrone [7].

Estrogen performs several essential functions in WAT, including promoting adipogenesis (differentiation of pre-adipocytes into mature adipocytes), modulating lipogenesis (storage of fatty acids) and influencing fat distribution. Reduced estrogen production in lipedemic adipocytes can lead to a decrease in healthy fat storage capacity, potentially resulting in hypertrophy of existing adipocytes and pathological fat accumulation [8].

In addition to aromatase, other steroidogenic enzymes in WAT include 17β-hydroxysteroid dehydrogenase (17β-HSD) and sulfotransferase (SULT1E1), which regulate the conversion and inactivation of estrogens. The activity of 17β-HSD, for example, controls the formation of estradiol from estrone, with a direct impact on the levels of active estrogen within adipose tissue. Changes in the activity of these enzymes can also influence the hormonal and metabolic picture in Lipedema.

Studies indicate that chronic inflammation associated with Lipedema can alter the expression of these enzymes, impacting both the production and inactivation of estrogens in WAT. Inflammatory cytokines can modify the expression of 17β-HSD and

SULT1E1, promoting an unfavorable environment for hormonal homeostasis. These enzymatic alterations can contribute to the progression of Lipedema, exacerbating fat deposition and promoting insulin resistance and local inflammation [9].

In addition to the direct impact on steroidogenic enzymes, inflammation and the altered hormonal environment in Lipedema can affect adipocyte function in other ways. The presence of chronic inflammation can promote the infiltration of immune cells, such as macrophages, into adipose tissue, further increasing the production of inflammatory cytokines and perpetuating a cycle of inflammation and metabolic dysfunction [10].

Intracrinology and estrogen metabolism in adipose tissue play crucial roles in the metabolic health and pathophysiology of Lipedema. Chronic inflammation associated with Lipedema can alter the expression and activity of steroidogenic enzymes in adipocytes, promoting a hormonal imbalance that exacerbates the condition. Understanding these mechanisms is fundamental to developing effective therapeutic strategies aimed at restoring hormonal homeostasis and improving metabolic health in patients with Lipedema.

In women with Lipedema, we know about the role of estrogen in the initiation and progression of the disease, but the vast majority of patients do not have abnormally high estrogen levels [11]. Several studies in the literature have shown that among the various abnormalities in the biological behavior of Lipedema adipocytes, the most noteworthy are increased expression of aromatases, among other enzymes involved in the synthesis of extra-gonadal steroids, and increased expression of inflammatory cytokines that induce changes in the expression of steroidogenesis enzymes, strongly suggesting that local estrogen production and metabolization in Lipedema adipose tissue play an important role in the disease [12].

Steroidogenesis in women's adipose tissue and intracrinology play key roles in regulating female sex hormones and maintaining hormonal health at different stages of a woman's life (**Figure 2**). The proper balance of these processes is essential for overall hormonal health and female well-being.

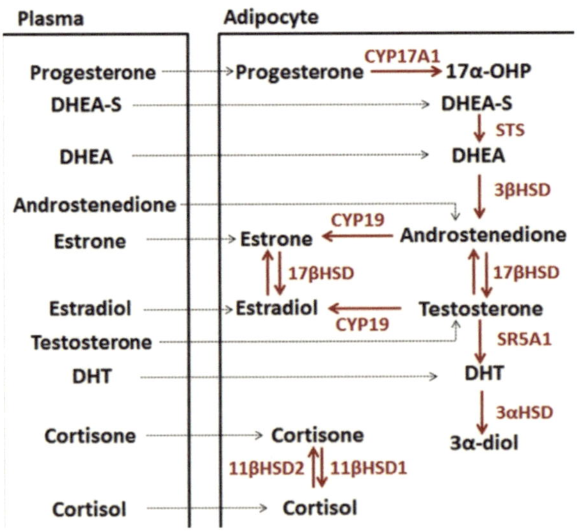

Figure 2.
Intracrinology Li et al. [13].

DOI: http://dx.doi.org/10.5772/intechopen.1006956

4. Aromatase expression in adipose tissue and Lipedema

Aromatase is a key enzyme in steroid metabolism that plays a significant role in modulating female sex hormones, such as estradiol, from androgen precursors in peripheral tissues, including adipose tissue. The expression of aromatase in adipose tissue throughout a woman's life plays a complex role in regulating fat distribution, metabolic function and the inflammatory response of this tissue.

During puberty, aromatase expression in adipose tissue is influenced by significant hormonal changes, such as increased estrogen levels. Aromatase converts testosterone into estradiol in adipocytes, impacting the differentiation and size of fat cells, as well as the distribution of body fat. Adequate levels of estradiol derived from aromatase expression in adipose tissue are essential for the regulation of lipid metabolism and energy storage during the development and maturation of adipose tissue.

During reproductive life, aromatase expression in adipose tissue maintains adequate estrogen levels for physiological processes such as the regulation of the menstrual cycle and the maintenance of metabolic function. Aromatase in adipocytes plays a role in regulating local steroidogenesis, influencing the production of other sex steroids and the inflammatory response in adipose tissue. Imbalances in aromatase expression can lead to changes in fat distribution, insulin resistance and chronic inflammation associated with metabolic and endocrine disorders such as metabolic syndrome.

During menopause, when estradiol levels decrease significantly, aromatase expression in adipose tissue may be compensatory as an attempt to maintain local estrogen levels. However, the limited ability of adipose tissue to compensate for estrogen deficiency during menopause can lead to changes in fat distribution, increased visceral adiposity and a higher risk of metabolic and cardiovascular complications [14].

The regulation of aromatase function in adipocytes is crucial for hormonal and metabolic homeostasis throughout a woman's life. In addition to directly influencing the production of estradiol and other sex steroids in adipose tissue, aromatase activity can also modulate the inflammatory response and cell proliferation in this tissue. Understanding the complex network of interactions between aromatase expression, local steroidogenesis and inflammation in adipose tissue is essential for developing effective therapeutic approaches to metabolic and endocrine disorders associated with female hormonal imbalance [15].

Aromatase overexpression in dysfunctional adipose tissue links obesity to postmenopausal breast cancer and would be a good example of the importance of local estrogen metabolism for women's health [16]. With that in mind, we could argue that metformin, as an aromatase inhibitor and insulin resistance agent, could have a role in the management of Lipedema, and for the future, it would be interesting to have more studies on this matter.

5. Role of estrogen in the biological behavior of adipose tissue Lipedema: understanding the possible pathways

Estrogen, a primary sex hormone in women, exerts its biological functions mainly through estrogen receptors, with the alpha-type estrogen receptor (ERα) being one of the most studied in this context.

Signaling via ERα is crucial in the regulation of adipogenesis. One prominent mechanism is the modulation of lipoprotein lipase (LPL), a key enzyme in the hydrolysis of triglycerides into free fatty acids and glycerol, processing the lipoproteins into fatty acids stored in adipose tissue. Studies show that activation of ERα reduces the activity, leading to less fat accumulation in adipocytes. This negative regulation is seen as a mechanism by which estrogen can help moderate the accumulation of body fat [17].

Another significant factor in estrogen-mediated adipogenesis is PPARγ (peroxisome proliferator-activated receptor gamma), a master regulator of adipocyte differentiation and the expression of genes involved in lipogenesis and fat storage. Estrogen signals and ERα activation appear to repress PPARγ activity, consequently inhibiting fat cell formation and fat accumulation [17].

Adrenergic receptors, specifically beta (β)-adrenergic receptors, are also influenced by estrogen signaling. They play an important role in lipolysis, the process of breaking down triglycerides into fatty acids and glycerol. Activation of ERα has been associated with modulation of the adrenergic response, possibly increasing the sensitivity of these receptors to stimulation, thus promoting lipolysis and a reduction in fat mass [18].

GLUT4 (glucose transporter type 4) is another critical component influenced by estrogen signaling. GLUT4 facilitates glucose uptake in adipose and muscle tissues. The regulation of GLUT4 through ERα may improve insulin sensitivity, increasing the glucose uptake by adipose cells and modulating energy storage [19].

In addition, estrogen can promote vasculogenesis and angiogenesis in adipose tissue through the induction of vascular endothelial growth factor (VEGF). This is essential for the expansion of adipose tissue, providing the nutrients and oxygen necessary for adipocyte growth. Evidence shows that alterations in serum VEGF and adipose tissue in women with Lipedema promote changes in local angiogenesis that seem to be directly associated with the progression of the disease [20].

The local estrogen load and the production of estrogens in specific tissues are regulated by enzymes such as aromatase, 17 beta-hydroxysteroid dehydrogenase (17β-HSD) and 3 beta-hydroxysteroid dehydrogenase (3β-HSD). Aromatase converts androgens into estrogens, while 17β-HSD and 3β-HSD regulate the conversion between estrogens and their metabolites. The activity of these enzymes can locally increase levels of estrogen levels, potentially influencing the development and function of adipocytes.

Therefore, estrogen and its signaling via ERα play multifaceted roles in the regulation of adipogenesis. Through the modulation of LPL, PPARγ, adrenergic receptors, GLUT4 and VEGF, and through the regulation of local estrogen synthesis enzymes such as aromatase, 17β-HSD and 3β-HSD, estrogen controls various aspects of fat storage and metabolism, possibly contributing to conditions of abnormal adipose tissue accumulation such as Lipedema. These insights highlight the complexity of female hormonal physiology, which involves not only ovarian production of hormones but also the inherent property of adipose tissue to carry out steroidogenesis—the magnitude of the impact of these locally produced hormones on women's health as a whole deserves our attention.

Female adipose tissue, modulating local estrogen production throughout a woman's reproductive milestones, contributes a large part of the total estrogen load, perhaps as much as the ovaries, and therefore, we cannot really understand female gonadal steroids without understanding adipose tissue.

Women's adipose tissue is a major endocrine organ and a reservoir for the synthesis of sex steroids, particularly estrogens.

6. Sex hormones, metabolic health and the regulation of fat distribution in women's lives

Now that we understand the contribution of adipose tissue to female hormonal health, we also need to understand how this impacts objectively on hormonal health and the distribution of body fat in women.

The behavior of adipose tissue in response to sex hormones, such as estradiol, testosterone and FSH (follicle-stimulating hormone), plays a critical role during women's reproductive milestones, such as menopause, pregnancy and puberty. These phases are marked by significant hormonal changes that influence the function and structure of adipose tissue, affecting fat distribution and female metabolic health [21].

Estradiol plays an important role in female metabolic health. Hormones help to integrate the metabolic interaction between major organs that are essential for intensive metabolic activities such as reproduction and metabolic function. Sex steroids are necessary to regulate the metabolism of adipocytes and also influence the remodeling of fat deposits. In humans, the factors that control fat distribution are partly determined by sex hormones.

During menopause, there is a drastic decrease in levels of estradiol, the main estrogen hormone, due to the cessation of ovarian function. With reduced estrogen levels, there is a change in the pattern of body fat distribution, with less fat being deposited in subcutaneous adipose tissue and an increase in visceral fat [22].

During pregnancy, dynamic hormonal changes occur, including a significant increase in estradiol and progesterone levels to sustain gestation. These hormones play an important role in regulating fat distribution during pregnancy, preparing maternal adipose tissue to store energy for lactation and fetal growth. Adipocytes respond to hormonal changes by increasing their lipid storage capacity, especially in the abdominal region and breasts, to support the energetic and physiological demands of pregnancy [23].

At puberty, hormonal fluctuations, including increased FSH levels, play an important role in the development of adipose tissue and fat distribution. FSH, along with other reproductive hormones, influences adipocyte maturation and can impact the amount and distribution of body fat. FSH receptors on adipocytes are involved in regulating fat cell differentiation and function, influencing the response of adipose tissue to hormonal changes characteristic of puberty [24].

In summary, the behavior of adipose tissue in response to sex hormones and FSH during menopause, pregnancy and puberty is fundamental to the regulation of fat distribution, metabolic function and overall health in women. Understanding these hormonal interactions is essential for addressing issues related to fertility, obesity, insulin resistance, cardiovascular disease and other conditions associated with hormonal imbalances throughout a woman's life.

7. Menopause and metabolic dysfunction associated with hypoestrogenism

Menopause and the end of reproductive life mark a period of significant transition in a woman's life, characterized by drastic hormonal changes that can impact metabolic health, insulin resistance, inflammation mechanisms and the behavior of adipose tissue. These changes have the potential to affect not only body composition and the associated risk of disease but also the progression of Lipedema. Although most women are diagnosed with Lipedema during their reproductive years, approximately 20% of women will be diagnosed during menopause and the vast majority of Lipedema sufferers experience a worsening of the condition during menopause [11].

With Lipedema being an estrogen-related disease that has been replicated for decades, it is not uncommon for menopausal women with Lipedema, despite being symptomatic, not to receive hormone therapy for fear of worsening Lipedema or even for their own doctors to contraindicate hormone therapy because of Lipedema. Neither option is correct, and both will harm the patient. Although very little has been published in the medical literature about HRT in women with menopausal Lipedema, what has been observed is that menopause and therefore hypoestrogenism do not improve Lipedema. On the contrary, many patients experience a worsening of the condition in this phase, not only because of the changes in the biological behavior of this diseased adipose tissue but also because of the systemic metabolic worsening that these patients will experience and which are typical of this phase: weight gain, visceral fat accumulation, insulin resistance, sleep disorders, HPA axis dysfunction, depression and anxiety [25].

Estrogen levels play a crucial role in determining the type of expansion and location of adipose tissue that changes as estrogen decreases due to medications, medical procedures and/or age. While normal estrogen levels result in hyperplastic growth of subcutaneous adipose tissue, reduced estrogen leads to hypertrophic expansion of metabolically harmful visceral adipose tissue [8].

During reproductive life, estrogen biosynthesis is carried out in a coordinated cyclical manner, particularly by the ovaries responding to ovarian gonadotropins. In addition, even before menopause, there is a small amount of steroids being produced in peripheral tissues, especially the woman's adipose tissue, also coordinated by pituitary gonadotrophins [26].

With menopause and the end of reproductive life, the ovaries cease to be the primary source of sex steroid synthesis and peripheral tissues take over. In addition, menopause also changes the expression and signaling of alpha and beta estrogen receptors in peripheral tissues, so that estrogen signaling in these tissues also changes with the onset of menopause [27].

In adipose tissue, in addition to the steroidogenesis responses coordinated by gonadotropins, there is a huge impact from the influence of inflammatory cytokines activating the expression of enzymes such as aromatase, sulfatases, 17 beta-hydroxysteroid dehydrogenase, 3 beta OH and 5 alpha reductase [28]. The influence of inflammation on the activity of these enzymes probably has a major impact on the synthesis of steroids, particularly estrogens, in the abnormally inflamed adipose tissue of Lipedema.

Insulin resistance, a metabolic imbalance characterized by the decreased effectiveness of insulin in reducing blood glucose levels, is a common complication associated with menopause and falling estrogen levels. Insulin resistance can lead to the accumulation of visceral fat, increased risk of type 2 diabetes and cardiovascular complications, contributing to an unfavorable metabolic profile in menopausal women [29].

With regard to adipose tissue, menopause can also induce changes in fat distribution, with a preferential shift from subcutaneous fat to visceral fat. Visceral adipose tissue is strongly associated with a higher risk of metabolic diseases, while subcutaneous adipose tissue has a more favorable metabolic profile. Therefore, fat redistribution during menopause may contribute to metabolic and cardiovascular complications in this period of a woman's life.

Women with Lipedema may experience increased discomfort and inflammation associated with the condition during menopause.

The drop in hormone levels, especially estrogen, can affect the inflammatory response in adipose tissue and the distribution of body fat, exacerbating the symptoms of Lipedema. In addition, insulin resistance and metabolic changes resulting from menopause can negatively impact the progression of Lipedema, increasing fat accumulation and inflammation in the affected tissues. Therefore, restricting estrogen therapy during menopause due to Lipedema has no biological plausibility.

On the other hand, it should be noted that poorly used estrogen therapy in women with Lipedema may contribute to worsening the condition—in this sense, it seems reasonable to avoid high doses, the oral route, which is generally associated with a worse estradiol/estrone ratio, and to make the necessary controls and adjustments to hormonal metabolomics, avoiding the formation of excess inflammatory estrones such as 16-oh-estrone in particular.

More studies are needed to define which type of hormone replacement should be most appropriate for menopausal women diagnosed with Lipedema: type of estrogen molecule, route of administration, maximum and minimum doses, hormone metabolomics adjustments as well as management of insulin resistance, inflammation, nutritional deficiencies, stress management, sleep and other factors that impact on the outcome of well-indicated hormone therapy with maximized benefits and minimized risks.

8. Thyroid hormones and adipose tissue

The International Lipedema Guideline published in 2021 recommends that every woman with Lipedema should undergo a detailed assessment of thyroid function, as it appears to be the most common hormonal dysfunction in women with Lipedema, affecting approximately 30% of women, with a prevalence above that of the general population [30].

Thyroid hormones play a crucial role in regulating the metabolism and function of adipocytes. The mechanism of action of these thyroid hormones directly influences metabolic activity, fat oxidation and adipocyte size [31]. In addition, the consensus itself suggests that the association with autoimmune thyroid disease (Hashimoto's thyroiditis) is common and that its investigation is therefore also necessary when Lipedema is diagnosed. It is known that the presence of thyroid autoimmunity per se is associated with higher levels of oxidative stress, regardless of the presence or absence of hypothyroidism da Silva [32].

It is currently understood that part of the process that initiates the thyroid autoimmunity process involves the interaction of a genetic risk associated with the presence of environmental triggers. Among the environmental triggers is the loss of selective intestinal permeability, called "leaky gut", which appears as one of the initial stages of the process that results in human autoimmunity [33]. This loss of the intestinal barrier generates chronic low-grade inflammation, partly due to the circulation of LPS (lipopolysaccharides) which, when circulating through the bloodstream, also reach the white adipocytes generating local inflammation, perhaps one of the main pathophysiological mechanisms of Lipedema [34].

TSH is produced by the pituitary gland and acts by stimulating the thyroid to release thyroid hormones such as T3. Once released by the thyroid, T3 exerts its effects by binding to specific nuclear receptors on target cells, such as white adipocytes. The activation of these receptors by T3 regulates genes involved in the regulation of metabolism and cell differentiation, directly influencing the function of adipocytes.

Thyroid hormones play a role in regulating lipolysis (breakdown of lipids) in adipocytes, stimulating the release of fatty acids and fat oxidation to provide the body with energy. In addition, T3 is known to influence insulin sensitivity and glucose metabolism in adipocytes, indirectly impacting fat storage and energy balance [31].

Thyroid hormones regulate adipocyte function primarily through T3 converted locally by the action of deiodinases, selenoproteases that mediate the peripheral conversion of T4 into T3. The peripheral conversion of t4 into t3 can suffer multiple interferences, which influence the activity of the deiodinases. The presence of local inflammation is known to reduce the conversion of T4 into T3, limiting the action of thyroid hormones in an inflammatory environment [35].

Evidence shows that there is an increased expression of inflammatory cytokines in lipedematous adipocytes [36], which suggests the possibility that local resistance to the action of thyroid hormones may develop in the adipose tissue of Lipedema, which in a way would further reduce the sensitivity of these cells to lipolytic stimuli and create an environment even more conducive to expansion and resistance to beta-oxidation [37].

Finally, it should also be noted that approximately 20% of patients with hypothyroidism have persistent complaints of hypothyroidism despite thyroid function being restored through hormone replacement that results in normalization of laboratory levels of thyroid function. Persistent symptoms include chronic fatigue, fluid retention and difficulty losing weight—symptoms that are also very common in women with Lipedema, suggesting that among women with Lipedema and hypothyroidism, there may be an overlap of complaints [38].

It is important to note that thyroid alterations in women with Lipedema can be both a cause and a consequence of the condition. For example, pre-existing thyroid dysfunction may predispose a woman to developing Lipedema due to the effects on adipocytes and lipid metabolism [39]. On the other hand, the abnormal accumulation of fat observed in Lipedema can lead to alterations in the regulation of thyroid hormones due to the influence of adipose tissue on thyroid activity, mainly through adipokines produced by adipose tissue such as leptin, which establishes communication between energy reserves in adipose tissue and the hypothalamic-pituitary-thyroid axis.

Finally, it is worth highlighting the impact of thyroid dysfunction on female fertility and gestational risks, which have already been well described in the literature [40]. The presence of anti-thyroid antibodies is related to lower ovarian reserve and worse gestational outcomes and a recent study highlighted an above population average prevalence of miscarriage in women with Lipedema, highlighting the need for these diagnoses to be made in all women seeking reproductive assistance [41].

9. Inflammation, LPS and estrogen metabolism

Chronic low-grade inflammation has been an important topic in recent medical research, especially in relation to the development and progression of metabolic diseases such as obesity and type 2 diabetes [42]. One of the underlying causes of this inflammation is the translocation of lipopolysaccharides (LPS), components of the outer membrane of gram-negative bacteria, from the intestine into the systemic circulation. This phenomenon can be amplified by increased intestinal permeability, often referred to as "leaky gut" [43].

LPS are components of the cell wall of gram-negative bacteria and, when translocated from the gut to the systemic circulation, can induce a significant inflammatory response. Increased intestinal permeability, often the result of dysbiosis or other intestinal barrier disorders, facilitates this translocation.

LPS are therefore endotoxins that, once in the bloodstream, can induce an innate immune response through the activation of Toll-like receptors (TLRs), particularly TLR4, on various cells in the body. In adipocytes or fat cells, this activation triggers a signaling cascade that results in the production of pro-inflammatory cytokines, such as tumor necrosis factor-alpha (TNF-α), interleukin-6 (IL-6) and interleukin-1 beta (IL-1β). Sustained elevation of these inflammatory mediators promotes a state of chronic low-grade inflammation [44].

This continuous inflammation also causes a change in the biological behavior of adipocytes. Firstly, it alters the ability of adipocytes to store lipids efficiently. Chronic inflammation disrupts the normal processes of lipogenesis and lipolysis, leading to the accumulation of free fatty acids in the blood, which can contribute to lipotoxicity in other organs. In addition, inflammation can interfere with insulin signaling in adipocytes, a crucial process for regulating glucose and lipid metabolism. Insulin resistance in adipocytes is characterized by a decrease in insulin-mediated glucose uptake, resulting in elevated blood glucose levels and contributing to hyperglycemia [45].

The pathophysiology of Lipedema remains largely unknown despite the advances made in recent years. Some points remain controversial, such as whether there is hypertrophy and/or hyperplasia of adipocytes, and whether there is thickening of the epidermis, among other controversial points from different studies. However, some other points seem to be less controversial, such as the presence of increased vascular permeability and fragility resulting in the accumulation of fluids and proteins in the affected areas and the malfunctioning of the lymphatic system early on in the disease [46].

But how and why does Lipedema begin? We know that there is a genetic predisposition and we understand that there is a huge influence of environmental and epigenetic factors, but in a disease with a prolonged and probably progressive evolution, the sooner we identify the factors that initiate and perpetuate the disease, the greater the chance of reducing its impact on patients' lives, including reducing its emotional and physical consequences and the total cost of treatment, which today ultimately falls on one or more expensive surgeries for health systems.

One of the hypotheses that has gained the most prominence is the influence of LPS in changing the biological behavior of white adipocytes [34].

We know that an imbalance of intestinal microbiota, associated with increased selective intestinal permeability (leaky gut), generates an increase in LPS and these LPS, produced at the intestinal level (metabolic endotoxemia), reach the white adipocytes generating an increase in inflammatory cytokines [47]. LPS modulates the functions of adipocytes directly through the activation of TLR-4 or indirectly, especially through the activation of macrophages, which in turn secrete cytokines that modulate the functions of adipocytes [48].

The gut microbiota plays a critical role in this process. Changes in the composition of the microbiome, caused by diet, antibiotic use or other factors, can influence the production of LPS and the integrity of the intestinal barrier. Therapeutic strategies aimed at restoring a healthy microbiota, such as the use of probiotics, prebiotics, exercise and proper diet, have shown a potential to decrease LPS translocation and reduce systemic inflammation [49].

In summary, chronic low-grade inflammation, fueled by intestinal lipopolysaccharide translocation, has profound effects on adipocyte function, disrupting lipid metabolism and insulin signaling, promoting insulin resistance and contributing to metabolic diseases. Understanding this complex mechanism offers avenues for therapeutic interventions aimed at mitigating inflammation and its metabolic consequences, not only in Lipedema but also in other comorbidities associated with Lipedema that are also linked to inflammation, LPS and endotoxemia, such as obesity (37 to 87%), hypothyroidism (31%), allergies and asthma (18%), PCOS (3 to 6%) and lymphedema [34].

In the context of Lipedema, this chronic inflammation perpetuated by LPS may aggravate the condition by interfering with normal WAT metabolism. Inflamed adipocytes not only contribute to insulin resistance, but also disrupt hormonal regulation, particularly in relation to local estrogen metabolism. White adipose tissue is not only an energy storage site, but also an important source of estrogen production, especially in post-menopausal women, where ovarian estrogen production is significantly reduced [50].

In white adipocytes, estrogens are produced from steroid precursors that arrive via the bloodstream, particularly androstenedione and testosterone through the action of the aromatase enzyme [8].

LPS-induced chronic inflammation can negatively affect aromatase expression and activity. Cytokines such as TNF-α and IL-6 are known to regulate aromatase expression, leading to altered estrogen production in adipose tissue, mainly through induction of the 4 OH estrone pathway [51]. This effect can have several negative consequences, including a hormonal imbalance which could, at least from a theoretical point of view, exacerbate the fat accumulation characteristic of Lipedema.

In addition, WAT dysfunction due to inflammation can promote an environment conducive to adipocyte hypertrophy and increase adipose tissue fibrosis. These factors further complicate the management of Lipedema, since fibrosis can hinder lymphatic drainage, aggravate edema and cause additional pain.

Therapeutic interventions aimed at restoring the integrity of the intestinal barrier by reducing LPS translocation may be a promising approach to mitigating chronic inflammation in Lipedema. Strategies such as modulation of the gut microbiome through probiotics, prebiotics and dietary changes, as well as the use of anti-inflammatory compounds, are being explored [52]. In addition, treatments that can positively regulate aromatase activity in WAT and restore estrogen balance may offer additional benefits in the management of Lipedema and consequently modulate inflammatory responses, adipocyte hyperplasia and hypertrophy, etc.

In summary, LPS-induced chronic inflammation appears to play an important role in the etiopathogenesis and progression of Lipedema, as well as influencing estrogen metabolism dysfunction in white adipose tissue. Understanding these mechanisms could open up new avenues for more effective treatments focused on both reducing inflammation and regulating hormones.

10. Closing remarks and future perspectives

The management of Lipedema, a condition characterized by the abnormal accumulation of fat in the lower body, is still evolving. Recent investigations suggest that aromatase inhibitors, insulin resistance regulators and anti-inflammatory agents could serve as promising therapeutic options.

Aromatase inhibitors (AIs), commonly used in the treatment of hormone-sensitive breast cancer, work by reducing estrogen levels. There is emerging evidence suggesting that estrogen may play a role in the pathogenesis of Lipedema due to its effects on adipocyte development and distribution. Some research indicates that estrogen sensitivity might exacerbate the condition, suggesting that AIs could alleviate symptoms by normalizing hormonal imbalances associated with Lipedema, however, normally, there is no serum estrogen excess detectable in women with Lipedema [53].

Insulin resistance is often observed in patients suffering from Lipedema and obesity, and tackling this aspect may be crucial for effective management. Medications such as metformin or even SGLT2 inhibitors may be plausible, which enhance insulin sensitivity, and may provide benefits not only in metabolic control but also potentially in reducing Lipedema-related symptoms. Research highlights the connections between insulin resistance and adipose tissue dysfunction, indicating that correcting these metabolic abnormalities could improve clinical outcomes in Lipedema [54]. On the other hand, women with Lipedema are normally exceptionally insulin sensitive, except when there is an association with obesity which is common but not a universal finding.

Furthermore, as for many means also an inflammatory disease, anti-inflammatory agents, including certain non-steroidal anti-inflammatory drugs (NSAIDs), anti-inflammatory diets and supplements, may address the chronic inflammation observed in individuals with Lipedema. As inflammation can exacerbate pain and discomfort, targeting this aspect could enhance the quality of life for patients [55].

In summary, targeting hormonal, metabolic and inflammatory pathways presents a multifaceted approach to the clinical management of Lipedema. Further research is warranted to establish the efficacy and safety of these therapeutic options in this specific patient population.

Lipedema is a complex disease that affects a high percentage of women: they will live their reproductive life with its challenges and struggles, contraception, pregnancy, postpartum, breastfeeding and finally menopause, and throughout their lives, they will have to deal with a pathology that in many ways is highly influenced by their hormones, particularly estrogens.

Author details

Juliana Bicca
Clinical Endocrinologist, Medical Director of Stonella Clinic, SP, Brazil

*Address all correspondence to: drajubicca@gmail.com

References

[1] Naaz A et al. Effect of ovariectomy on adipose tissue of mice in the absence of estrogen receptor alpha (ERα): A potential role for estrogen receptor beta (ERβ). Hormone and Metabolic Research. 2002;**34**(11/12):758-763

[2] Kissebah AH, Evans DJ, Peiris A, Wilson CR, Vague J, Björntorp P, et al. Metabolic Complications of Human Obesities. Amsterdam: Excerpta Medica; 1985. p. 115

[3] Connolly S. Does lipoedema mimic pregnancy? Journal of Lymphoedema. 2022;**17**(1):19

[4] Lassek WD, Gaulin SJC. Waist-hip ratio and cognitive ability: Is gluteofemoral fat a privileged store of neurodevelopmental resources? Evolution and Human Behavior. 2008;**29**(1):26-34. ISSN 1090-5138. DOI: 10.1016/j.evolhumbehav.2007.07.005

[5] Carré N, Binart N. Prolactin and adipose tissue. Biochimie. 2014;**97**:16-21

[6] Straub RH. The complex role of estrogens in inflammation. Endocrine Reviews. 2007;**28**(5):521-574

[7] Hetemäki N et al. Adipose tissue estrogen production and metabolism in premenopausal women. The Journal of Steroid Biochemistry and Molecular Biology. 2021;**209**:105849

[8] Steiner BM, Berry DC. The regulation of adipose tissue health by estrogens. Frontiers in Endocrinology. 2022;**13**:889923

[9] Bornstein SR, Rutkowski H, Vrezas I. Cytokines and steroidogenesis. Molecular and Cellular Endocrinology. 2004;**215**(1-2):135-141

[10] Schäffler A, Schölmerich J. Innate immunity and adipose tissue biology. Trends in Immunology. 2010;**31**(6):228-235

[11] Patton L et al. Observational study on a large Italian population with lipedema: Biochemical and hormonal profile, anatomical and clinical evaluation, self-reported history. International Journal of Molecular Sciences. 2024;**25**(3):1599

[12] Bauer A-T et al. Adipose stem cells from lipedema and control adipose tissue respond differently to adipogenic stimulation in vitro. Plastic and Reconstructive Surgery. 2019;**144**(3):623-632

[13] Li J, Papadopoulos V, Vihma V. Steroid biosynthesis in adipose tissue. Steroids. 2015;**103**:89-104. ISSN 0039-128X. DOI: 10.1016/j.steroids.2015.03.016

[14] Bulun SE, Zeitoun K, Sasano H, Simpson ER. Aromatase in aging women. Semin Reprod Endocrinol. 1999;**17**(4):349-358. DOI: 10.1055/s-2007-1016244. PMID: 10851574

[15] Wang X, Simpson ER, Brown KA. Aromatase overexpression in dysfunctional adipose tissue links obesity to postmenopausal breast cancer. The Journal of Steroid Biochemistry and Molecular Biology. 2015;**153**:35-44

[16] Price TM et al. Estrogen regulation of adipose tissue lipoprotein lipase—Possible mechanism of body fat distribution. American Journal of Obstetrics and Gynecology. 1998;**178**(1):101-107

[17] Yoon M. The role of PPARα in lipid metabolism and obesity: Focusing on the effects of estrogen on PPARα

actions. Pharmacological Research. 2009;**60**(3):151-159

[18] Kuryłowicz A. Estrogens in adipose tissue physiology and obesity-related dysfunction. Biomedicine. 2023;**11**(3):690

[19] Fatima LA et al. Estradiol stimulates adipogenesis and Slc2a4/GLUT4 expression via ESR1-mediated activation of CEBPA. Molecular and Cellular Endocrinology. 2019;**498**:110447

[20] Felmerer G et al. Increased levels of VEGF-C and macrophage infiltration in lipedema patients without changes in lymphatic vascular morphology. Scientific Reports. 2020;**10**(1):10947

[21] Wells JCK. Sexual dimorphism of body composition. Best Practice & Research Clinical Endocrinology & Metabolism. 2007;**21**(3):415-430

[22] Lizcano F, Guzmán G. Estrogen deficiency and the origin of obesity during menopause. BioMed Research International. 2014;**2014**(1):757461

[23] Kinoshita T, Itoh M. Longitudinal variance of fat mass deposition during pregnancy evaluated by ultrasonography: The ratio of visceral fat to subcutaneous fat in the abdomen. Gynecologic and Obstetric Investigation. 2006;**61**(2):115-118

[24] Loomba-Albrecht LA, Styne DM. Effect of puberty on body composition. Current Opinion in Endocrinology, Diabetes and Obesity. 2009;**16**(1):10-15

[25] Ou Y-J et al. Association between menopause, postmenopausal hormone therapy and metabolic syndrome. Journal of Clinical Medicine. 2023;**12**(13):4435

[26] Savolainen-Peltonen H et al. Estrogen biosynthesis in breast adipose tissue during menstrual cycle in women with and without breast cancer. Gynecological Endocrinology. 2018;**34**(12):1039-1043

[27] Anwar A et al. Site-specific regulation of oestrogen receptor-α and-β by oestradiol in human adipose tissue. Diabetes, Obesity and Metabolism. 2001;**3**(5):338-349

[28] Simpson ER. Sources of estrogen and their importance. The Journal of Steroid Biochemistry and Molecular Biology. 2003;**86**(3-5):225-230

[29] Genazzani A, Petrillo T, Semprini E, Aio C, Foschi M, Ambrosetti F, et al. Metabolic syndrome, insulin resistance and menopause: The changes in body structure and the therapeutic approach. GREM Gynecological and Reproductive Endocrinology & Metabolism. 2024:086-091. DOI: 10.53260/grem.234026

[30] Herbst KL et al. Standard of care for lipedema in the United States. Phlebology. 2021;**36**(10):779-796

[31] Obregon M-J. Adipose tissues and thyroid hormones. Frontiers in Physiology. 2014;**5**:479

[32] Silva D, Bruno G, Yamauchi MA, Bagatini MD. Oxidative stress in Hashimoto's thyroiditis: Possible adjuvant therapies to attenuate deleterious effects. Molecular and Cellular Biochemistry. 2023;**478**(4):949-966

[33] Zhu X et al. Intestinal microbiota regulates the gut-thyroid axis: The new dawn of improving Hashimoto thyroiditis. Clinical and Experimental Medicine. 2024;**24**(1):39

[34] Kruglikov IL, Scherer PE. Is the endotoxin-complement cascade the major driver in lipedema? Trends in Endocrinology and Metabolism. Sep 2024;**35**(9):769-780. DOI: 10.1016/j.

tem.2024.04.004. PMID: 38688780; PMCID: PMC11387139 [Epub 2024 Apr 29]

[35] AL-Ghadban S et al. Dilated blood and lymphatic microvessels, angiogenesis, increased macrophages, and adipocyte hypertrophy in lipedema thigh skin and fat tissue. Journal of Obesity. 2019;**2019**(1):8747461

[36] Wolf S et al. A distinct cytokine profile and stromal vascular fraction metabolic status without significant changes in the lipid composition characterizes lipedema. International Journal of Molecular Sciences. 2021;**22**(7):3313

[37] Mancini A et al. Thyroid hormones, oxidative stress, and inflammation. Mediators of Inflammation. 2016;**2016**(1):6757154

[38] Wiersinga WM. T4+ T3 combination therapy: An unsolved problem of increasing magnitude and complexity. Endocrinology and Metabolism. 2021;**36**(5):938-951

[39] Sesmilo G et al. Role of thyroid hormones on serum leptin levels. European Journal of Endocrinology. 1998;**139**(4):428-430

[40] Wang R et al. Autoimmune thyroid disease and ovarian hypofunction: A review of literature. Journal of Ovarian Research. 2024;**17**(1):125

[41] Hasegawa Y et al. Effect of hypothyroidism and thyroid autoimmunity on the ovarian reserve: A systematic review and meta-analysis. Reproductive Medicine and Biology. 2022;**21**(1):e12427

[42] Lee YS, Olefsky J. Chronic tissue inflammation and metabolic disease. Genes & Development. 2021;**35**(5-6):307-328

[43] Page MJ, Kell DB, Pretorius E. The role of lipopolysaccharide-induced cell signalling in chronic inflammation. Chronic Stress. 2022;**6**:24705470221076390

[44] Okla M et al. Inhibitory effects of toll-like receptor 4, NLRP3 inflammasome, and interleukin-1β on white adipocyte browning. Inflammation. 2018;**41**:626-642

[45] Moreno-Navarrete JM et al. A role for adipocyte-derived lipopolysaccharide-binding protein in inflammation- and obesity-associated adipose tissue dysfunction. Diabetologia. 2013;**56**:2524-2537

[46] Buck DW et al. Lipedema: A relatively common disease with extremely common misconceptions. Plastic and Reconstructive Surgery–Global Open. 2016;**4**(9):e1043

[47] Salguero MV et al. Dysbiosis of gram-negative gut microbiota and the associated serum lipopolysaccharide exacerbates inflammation in type 2 diabetic patients with chronic kidney disease. Experimental and Therapeutic Medicine. 2019;**18**(5):3461-3469

[48] Munro P et al. Modulation of the inflammatory response to LPS by the recruitment and activation of brown and brite adipocytes in mice. American Journal of Physiology-Endocrinology and Metabolism. 2020;**319**(5):E912-E922

[49] Grylls A, Seidler K, Neil J. Link between microbiota and hypertension: Focus on LPS/TLR4 pathway in endothelial dysfunction and vascular inflammation, and therapeutic implication of probiotics. Biomedicine & Pharmacotherapy. 2021;**137**:111334

[50] Cawthorn WP, Sethi JK. TNF-α and adipocyte biology. FEBS Letters. 2008;**582**(1):117-131

[51] Salama SA et al. Effect of tumor necrosis factor-α on estrogen metabolism and endometrial cells: Potential physiological and pathological relevance. The Journal of Clinical Endocrinology & Metabolism. 2009;**94**(1):285-293

[52] Li X, Hu D, Tian Y, Song Y, Hou Y, Sun L, et al. Protective effects of a novel Lactobacillus rhamnosus strain with probiotic characteristics against lipopolysaccharide-induced intestinal inflammation in vitro and in vivo. Food & Function. 22 Jul 2020;**11**(7):5799-5814. DOI: 10.1039/d0fo00308e. PMID: 32568317

[53] Al-Ghadban S, Teeler ML, Bunnell BA. Estrogen as a Contributing Factor to the Development of Lipedema [Internet]. Hot Topics in Endocrinology and Metabolism. London, UK: IntechOpen; 2021. DOI: 10.5772/intechopen.96402

[54] Poojari A, Dev K, Rabiee A. Lipedema: Insights into morphology, pathophysiology, and challenges. Biomedicine. 2022;**10**(12):3081

[55] Kruppa P et al. Lipedema stage affects adipocyte hypertrophy, subcutaneous adipose tissue inflammation and interstitial fibrosis. Frontiers in Immunology. 2023;**14**:1223264